ONE FAILURE AT A TIME
A MODERN SURVIVAL GUIDE

SUZANNA ALSAYED

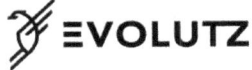

Copyright © 2024 by Suzanna Alsayed

All rights reserved. No part of this publication may be reproduced, distributed, or transmitted in any form or by any means, including photocopying, recording, or other electronic or mechanical methods, without the prior written permission of the publisher, except in the case of brief quotations embodied in critical reviews and certain other non-commercial uses permitted by copyright law.

This is a true story based on actual events and experiences. The individuals, places, and incidents portrayed herein are derived from authentic historical records, interviews, and personal accounts. To protect the identities of those involved, all names have been changed. The author has made every effort to faithfully recreate the essence and authenticity of the events while respecting the privacy and confidentiality of the real individuals. Every effort has been made to accurately and legally depict the events and circumstances surrounding the individuals involved.

The publisher, author, and editors have taken great care to ensure that all information presented in this book is accurate and reliable. However, they make no representations or warranties regarding the completeness or accuracy of the contents. The publisher and author shall not be held liable for any errors or omissions in this work or for any damages arising from using this information.

ISBN 978-1-7380736-2-7 (paperback)
ISBN 978-1-7380736-0-3 (hardcover)
ISBN 978-1-7380736-1-0 (eBook)

Cover design: bmcdesign & Suzanna Alsayed
Interior design: Amber Helt, Rooted in Writing LLC
Structural editor: Dragan Vukicevic
Editor: Maya Berger, What I Mean To Say
Editor: Kate McCandless, MLIS
Editor: Rachel Small, Rachel Small Editing

www.evolutz.com

DISCLAIMER #1: This book is not a replacement for professional help, such as psychotherapy, mental health counseling, or financial, legal, or other professional services. This is an inspirational self-help book on navigating life (based on my personal experiences) and its different obstacles. If you require professional help, please contact a specialist or professional.

DISCLAIMER #2: The individuals mentioned in this book are only included to contribute to the narrative's authenticity and depth. However, it is crucial to note that the portrayal of individuals is based on the author's perspective and interpretation of events. Every effort has been made to maintain privacy and confidentiality and avoid defamatory content.

The author does not endorse or encourage any harmful or libelous actions toward individuals mentioned in the book. The book aims to share experiences, insights, and personal growth journeys respectfully and responsibly.

It is important to approach the information presented in this book with an open mind, recognizing that each person's experiences and perceptions may differ. The reader is encouraged to exercise their own judgment and discretion when interpreting and applying the information to their own lives.

The author and publisher disclaim any liability for any offense, harm, or misunderstanding arising from the interpretation or application of the content in this book. This disclaimer is intended to protect the rights, privacy, and well-being of the individuals mentioned and ensure a responsible and respectful portrayal of their stories.

CONTENT WARNING:
This book addresses sensitive topics.

I believe in providing a safe reading experience, so please be aware that this book refers to and explores themes that may be distressing or triggering for some readers, including the following:

Abandonment; animal distress; body image; COVID-19 pandemic; grief and loss; immigration; marriage and divorce; mental health; racism and discrimination; war, violence, and terrorism; and women's reproductive health.

Some of these themes are integral to the story and may evoke strong emotions. If you feel that any of them may be triggering for you, consider pausing before engaging or re-engaging with this content and/or seek support from friends, family, or mental health professionals.

Your comfort level is important to me. Please enjoy the book at your own pace.

To Babyshka

CONTENTS

Enigmatic – Unlocking the Unknown   1

CHAPTER I
Sisu: A Tale of Nostalgia   9

CHAPTER II
Hiraeth: Echoes of the Past   43

CHAPTER III
Steadfast: Unwavering Amid Change   61

CHAPTER IV
Epiphany: Embracing the Shadows   87

CHAPTER V
Lamentation: The Unveiled Cycle   111

CHAPTER VI
Forelsket: The Spellbinding Waltz   133

CHAPTER VII
Serendipity: Embracing the Rhythm of Life   147

Navīna Ātman: Unearthing Inner Evolution   165

Acknowledgments   171

Notes   173

INTRODUCTION

~~ENIGMATIC:~~ UNLOCKING THE UNKNOWN

["Enigmatic": adjective / e-(ˌ)nig-ˈma-tik/]
Of, relating to, or resembling an enigma: mysterious.[1]

COMPARED TO SOME, I have lived at a fast pace. I have been fortunate enough to have gathered experiences that have allowed me to reflect, make risky yet beneficial decisions, and build the kind of life I always imagined for myself.

I believe in doing the right thing and have dedicated myself to sharing the lessons I have learned throughout my journey. I always wanted to write a book, even if I did not have a story that went viral. Instead, I have a real-life narrative with real-life lessons that anyone, regardless of age, race, gender, or other characteristics, can benefit from and apply.

I am just like you.

What solidified my decision to write this book was a quote often attributed to Brené Brown: "One day, you will tell your story of how you overcame what you went through, and it will become someone else's survival guide."[2] Well, *One Failure at a Time* is my modern survival guide. I believe this book has the potential to assist individuals in assessing their current situations and extracting valuable lessons from any challenges, confusion, or misinformation that piqued their curiosity and led them to pick up this book.

Whatever you are going through, I want you to know that your feelings are valid, and you might be taking the first step toward self-discovery. While this book will not sugarcoat anything, it will guide you through a process of reflection and realization.

Whether we like it or not, we humans have a lot to learn, and we often have a great deal of trauma, hurt, and fear to address and heal from. This modern survival guide is here to help shed light on these topics.

One Failure at a Time will cover the elements of organic personal growth. While reading, you might question what you already know (or thought you knew) about your relationships, friendships, influences in your environment, and general approach to life. I have made it my mission to understand why certain events unfolded as they did for me and where I have fallen short. That mission has changed my life.

The book will encompass a wide range of topics, including romantic relations, our bonds with friends, parents, siblings, acquaintances, and, perhaps most crucially, our relationship with ourselves. Many factors impact the success of our connections, such as our cultural awareness and how that shapes us, our responses to the words and actions of others, and our ethics. These elements can affect how we choose partners, process information, and understand loss, death, hope, and love.

Patterns will repeat themselves until we take the time to understand what they are trying to teach us. Only once we learn, forgive ourselves, surrender, and come to peace with everything will we be able to move forward.

We are often not taught these basic principles, especially when it comes to intimate relationships. We then wonder why we chose the wrong partners and are unhappy in our current relationships. Yet, we might or are compelled to present these relationships as picture-perfect on social media—but, let's be honest, picture-perfect does not exist and usually is not the reality behind closed doors.

I am not a conspiracist, but from my experience, the Western educational, economic, and cultural systems, on top of the social norms that so many of us are raised in, arguably focus on scaring or "controlling" young people. We are encouraged to go to school, then to college or university (where we often accumulate debt), get married, have kids, get a job, and work on our retirement plan. Once we retire, only then can we begin to live and enjoy our lives. However, this formula does not account for unexpected hardships, sicknesses, and death. Life is a revolving door of people and circumstances, and the door can close on our lives sooner than we expect.

I bought into that system; I went to school, got married, had a beautiful house and a good job, and did everything right. I had completed the "American dream" checklist, played by the rules, and accomplished everything I had planned before turning twenty-five. I could have been considered a success story. I should have been proud, but instead, I was miserable. I just wanted to run away and restart. And that's precisely what I did once I recognized that I had been living my life based on the influence of others.

That's when the real tests entered my life.

In her book *Becoming*, Michelle Obama discusses the notion of living life via a checklist. She reflects on how societal expectations often lead us to pursue predefined goals and achievements, to tick off items on a checklist of what we believe we should do. She writes that it's important to question whether these goals truly align with our desires and aspirations. Obama encourages her readers to focus on discovering their own passions, values, and purpose rather than blindly following societal norms or external expectations.[3]

Likewise, in this book, I aim to inspire you to leap and follow your own path, one that can activate an unexpected awakening within you.

One thing that often stops us from taking a leap of faith is the fear of failure. But what I want you to understand while you read this book and are processing whatever you are going through is that failure is inevitable, suffering is predestined, and heartbreak is unavoidable.[4] To complicate things further, even though many of us dread failure, we can also fear success—it's a double-edged sword. Being successful (whatever success means to you) can be frightening because it requires sacrifice, time, and commitment.

I simply assume that you are going through something. Because there has not been a day in my life or my friends' lives where we weren't surprised with lemons; in turn, we had to find a way to make lemonade or continually refine its recipe.[5]

Life does not get easier. Problems will always be present no matter what you do, and old problems get replaced by new ones.[6] The goal in life should not be to get rid of problems but to become a chameleon and adapt when they appear. How you perceive and respond to these problems will make a difference in your life. And ever so often, life tests you to the extreme, presenting situations and questions without easy answers. Otherwise, why would you be here, flipping through the pages of this book?

Anything that we will choose in life will be hard. Everything requires sacrifice, commitment, and being true to the life that you want to live. *Life is hard—at the end of the day, you must choose.* Only when you are ready to evaluate your values, behaviors, and habits will you begin to create powerful and effective change for yourself.

We are all full of excuses until we decide that we deserve better. Someone can tell you a million times that you're worth more than what you're currently getting out of life, but you'll only believe it once you realize it on your own. Everything comes from within; once you accept that, your journey can begin. It is never too late to start or end things, to reexamine your conditioned responses and reconsider what you value and how you measure personal and professional failures and successes.

Self-discovery and healing does not happen overnight, though. It requires dedication, discipline, consistency, and the will to be vulnerable with yourself and others. When you open yourself to this process, one of the main things you may discover is childhood traumas and how they have shaped your everyday life, reactions, and choices.

Understanding your emotions, responses, needs, wants, and dreams is crucial because no one else can ever fully understand how you feel. Nobody has that ability because nobody is you. No one will truly get it, no matter how often and diligently you explain yourself or try to describe or script your feelings.

Even though no one can ever know you the way you know yourself, at the end of the day, we all worry about the same things: money, work, family, relationships, and health, but these elements can impact us in different phases of our lives. Hence, the difference between our healed and unhealed selves is in how we react to our trials.

The good news is that our problems are common.

We are not special;[7] we are just sometimes misguided.

My desire to press the restart button on my entire life prompted me to tell my story. I wish I had been exposed to a book like this when I was younger; it might have guided and saved me from many heartbreaks and meltdowns and from feeling misunderstood and blamed. It would have helped me focus more on my priorities and beliefs.

Each chapter will cover different phases and events in my life where I learned hard lessons that changed my future. To add additional value, my personal stories are backed up with research, best practices, tips, and facts.

Chapter 1 introduces my family's immigration story, and I explore the coping mechanisms I developed to navigate my challenges. I describe how my parents' high expectations compelled me to conform to societal and cultural norms early in life, which later ignited a desire to uncover the path to authentic living. This chapter also heavily focuses on theory to arm you with concepts and avenues to which you might not have been exposed before.

In Chapter 2, I explore how living in a foreign country introduced abandonment issues into my life. I also reveal how, amid these challenges, I discovered a source of nurturing love from a special individual. Reflecting on the impressionable nature of childhood, I investigate how early experiences shape our perspectives on the world and the people around us.

By Chapter 3, I already feel as if I have lived multiple lifetimes—from becoming a professional athlete to training in the circus, playing chess competitively, and trying to become a dancer and actor in New York. I was just a teenager trying to find my way in life, but I learned the most important lesson: the power of consistency and discipline.

In Chapters 4 and 5, I look at the impact of my culture, early influences, and expectations on my adult relationships. I examine how the intricate interplay of female and masculine energies shapes our daily habits and dynamics within relationships. These chapters emphasize the importance of self-care and self-worth because putting ourselves first is the key to cultivating genuine self-love and inner strength, regardless of our circumstances.

In Chapter 6, a glimmer of hope emerges. I saw potential for positive change ahead; yet, I soon realized that my growth had only just begun, with more lessons waiting for me. I learned the art of survival and gained perspective, inching closer to a place where I could breathe freely once more. This chapter reminds us that a single moment can reshape our entire lives.

In Chapter 7, my journey comes full circle. After a decade of self-discovery, I embraced life with all its complexities and finally saw the sweet rewards of all the hard work and dedication I had invested in myself.

I hope reading this book will make you feel seen and understood, giving you the courage and knowledge you need to begin your inner work and uncover your full potential.

1

SISU: A TALE OF NOSTALGIA

["Sisu": noun / see'-soo/]
Strength of will, determination, perseverance, and acting rationally in the face of adversity.[1]

AS I SIT POUNDING AWAY at my keyboard, I reflect on how I escaped the nostalgia trap. It's been a long and winding road, but I'm here, ready to share my experiences, theories, and life in the hopes of helping you navigate your path.

What I mean by "the nostalgia trap" is the tendency to romanticize past events and experiences, which often prevents us from living in the moment and moving forward.

For many of us, the past can be a source of comfort and familiarity, representing a time when things were known and predictable. Looking back can evoke strong feelings of nostalgia, especially when we associate memories with positive experiences or significant relationships, leading us to dwell on them and yearn for that sense of happiness we once experienced. By contrast, the present and future are often filled with uncertainty and change, and revisiting the past can be a way to avoid facing the unknown. We all fall victim to the nostalgia trap at times.

It's easy to get sentimental about the events in our lives, no matter who we are or what we've been through.

I'll be the first to admit that I'm a sentimental person. I love to write, reread, and collect old journals, letters, notes, and plane tickets, and I also develop photos to make photo albums. These personal archives serve as a tangible reminder of how far I've come and how much I've grown. But getting to this point was challenging. I had to go through many redirections and much uncertainty and self-doubt to acquire the peace and fulfillment I have today.

It wasn't until I analyzed the events in my life, a process I document in this book, that I realized I had been romanticizing my past. I discovered that I had idealized certain notions and aspirations I'd had, believing they were the key to happiness. My desire to make my parents proud led me to glamorize my every achievement, convinced that their love was tied to my success. Similarly, I strived to become a professional athlete and an exceptional student, convinced that this would validate my worth. I ended up painting a picture of the future in my head—a loving marriage, wonderful children, a big home, and a seemingly flawless existence as a career-driven woman, ideal wife, and nurturing mother. Sounds perfect, right?

Societal pressures, my parents, and the people around me had ingrained these ideals into my psyche, and I had fully bought into them. I equated perfection with happiness, believing that fulfilling society's expectations would lead to a fulfilled life.

It turns out I was wrong, and in this chapter, I'll share how I slowly came to that realization. I hope doing so will encourage you to embark on your own introspection and arrive at your own conclusions.

We must start at the beginning, where the foundations of my life were laid. As I mentioned in the introduction, this chapter offers more theoretical knowledge than later ones, setting the stage before looking at my personal experiences in more depth. I urge you to take the time to understand this groundwork; it will help you gain insights and make connections as you progress through the rest of the chapters.

A CHILD OF IMMIGRANTS

Our formative years shape who we become, and through introspection, we can revisit past events, the decisions that were made, and the circumstances that influenced them, in turn, allowing us to gain a deeper understanding of ourselves and our patterns.

So, let's start from the beginning.

My parents were immigrants, which meant they had to work hard, make countless sacrifices, and endure unfair treatment that often went unnoticed by others. As a child, I witnessed firsthand my parents' struggles, from the language barriers and discrimination to the financial burdens and cultural adjustments. Yet, despite all these challenges, they never gave up and continued to fight for a better life.

But let's be honest: many immigrant parents are a different breed. They're often harder on their kids, more demanding, and less forgiving. It can be easy to feel as if our parents don't understand us or are pushing us too hard. It might seem as though they're being cruel when they've just been through hell and back and want their children to succeed where they couldn't.[2] They want us to have the opportunities they never had, to live the lives they dreamed of living. For many children of immigrant parents, the pressure to succeed can be suffocating. And my parents fell into that category since they wanted me to be the best, thrive, and fully live the "American dream."

It's a noble ambition, but it can have unintended long-term consequences.

Honestly, for many years, I was upset with my parents for being strict, demanding, and traditional. If you're like me, appreciating this approach may take a while. It took me almost twenty-five years. My parents survived unimaginable hardships and wanted me to triumph because they know what it takes to make it in this world.

Yet, even with all the appreciation you might gain over time, it is crucial to recognize that some of your parents' behaviors may have been inexcusable, whether they were immigrants or not. You have every right to feel how you feel or felt, and it is necessary to understand how their actions may have influenced and created patterns in your life.

To this day, I occasionally struggle to communicate and find common ground with my parents. But I understand that everything they've done has been a product of their circumstances. They came from a different world, time, and culture, and they've given everything to create a new life for their children. It's a debt that can never be fully repaid but can be honored by learning and accepting.

Being an immigrant in a new country is tough. You're isolated from your family and friends and trying to navigate a new culture, language, and social norms. The pressure to provide for your family while trying to assimilate into a foreign land and build a support system can be enough to make anyone buckle under it.[3]

As someone who witnessed it directly through my parents, I know that the psychological toll of immigration can be immense. Although my parents were considered adults when they had me, they were young adults, and their experiences growing up in different cultures affected how they raised my sister and me. My father lived through several wars in the Middle East, and my mother grew up in the former USSR. During the 1990s, the conditions in Eurasia and the Middle East were far from ideal, prompting my parents to make the big decision to establish a new home across the ocean.

Around the time my parents received the necessary paperwork and approval for migration, my father was offered a full scholarship to stay and train as a cardiovascular surgeon, placing him at a crossroads. Remaining in his home country to pursue his studies would have assured him a prosperous individual future. On the other hand, declining the scholarship for relocation meant re-establishing his credibility in a foreign country, but this option held the potential for a brighter future for his family.

Ultimately, he chose the latter path.

My father once confessed, "My dream had always been to become a cardiovascular surgeon, but I couldn't allow myself to be selfish. So, I relinquished my dream for a grander vision. I knew the road ahead would be strewn with challenges and personal sacrifices, but I was willing to endure it all for my family's well-being. I had faith that I would eventually accomplish my true calling."

My parents thus found themselves in the Western world in their mid-twenties trying to create a better life for themselves and their children. However, the weight of their past experiences made it hard for them to adapt to their new environment and often affected their mental and physical health.

To make things even more difficult, my parents' degrees were invalid in their new country. My dad, a medical doctor, had to redo his studies, while my mom, a civil engineer, had to switch careers entirely. Making ends meet was a perpetual battle, especially in those early years.

My father has often recounted the struggles he faced to secure a spot as a student or attain employment at any level. Despite possessing the qualifications of a skilled doctor, with a degree completed with excellence, and a history of prior work experience across various countries, he encountered major challenges. As a foreigner, he found that his international experiences held little weight in the eyes of Western employers or academic institutions—not to mention the regulatory barriers he had to overcome to be a recognized practitioner.

My father also endured blatant discrimination within the universities. Even after achieving the highest grades, passing all the foreign medical exams available, and converting his qualifications to a new system, he was relegated to waiting lists year after year. He was strung along in this disheartening way for three long years, only to be informed that there was no record of his application. This was later rectified when my father showed proof of admission, but it didn't change the outcome.

While he was getting nowhere academically, my father, willing to work any hours, applied for jobs, including one as a pizza delivery driver since he already had a car and a valid driver's license. However, he was continually turned away due to his perceived lack of local experience.

I often reflect on the despair he must have felt during that time. The constant barrage of rejections takes a toll, particularly when one is responsible for supporting a family.

Eventually, my dad landed a job as a dishwasher at a Middle Eastern restaurant. I still remember him coming home wearing shoes three sizes too big because he couldn't afford ones that fit. He had to stuff them with socks to keep them on while he washed dishes, the water dripping down and soaking his feet.

Meanwhile, my mom was almost always home alone, caring for a toddler and a newborn.

My father was grateful for securing temporary employment, although his work environment was toxic. The employers' behavior was demeaning, and they ridiculed him for working as a dishwasher. They would snap their fingers and call, "Doctor, come here and fetch us a glass of water." Given the responsibility of providing for our family, my father felt compelled to endure these degrading remarks in silence.

However, between the discrimination he faced throughout his three-year quest for medical school admission and the challenges at his job, my father reached a breaking point. At that time, his only valuable possession was a car valued at $4,500.00. Seeking a way out, he approached a dealership; they offered him $1,350.00 for the car, and he accepted the offer.

My father's patience was exhausted, and he had limited options: one, continue working in the same place, or, two, try somewhere else. Armed with the proceeds from selling the car, and despite knowing little English, he purchased a cross-country bus ticket, fueled by the hope of a brighter future for his family.

The journey was long, and my father reached his destination late at night. Upon arriving at the apartment he'd rented, he found only a metal bed frame and a solitary chair. In lieu of a proper sleeping arrangement, he draped his coat over the frame's metal railings and managed to get some rest. This makeshift arrangement continued for a few days until he finally had the means to purchase a mattress.

Thankfully, my dad quickly secured a job at a bakery, working shifts lasting twelve to twenty-four hours, earning $5.00 per hour in cash. With this demanding routine, he didn't have the time nor resources to attend English classes; instead, he would borrow English dictionaries from the library then write a dozen new words on his hands and arms each day and practice them during his long work hours. This marked the humble beginning of my father's more-formal English-language education.

What I've shared with you here merely skims the surface of my parents' challenges during their immigration. I wanted to provide a glimpse into their life during their mid-twenties, when their survival instincts peaked. My family often talks about my father's favorite film, *The Pursuit of Happyness*.[4] The bathroom scene, when Will Smith's character embraces his son, resonates deeply with me, and every time I watch it, I'm overcome with emotion. As a child, I witnessed the desperation in my parents' eyes and shared similar tearful moments with them in the face of adversity.

I've come to understand the nuances of my parents' immigration experience and the reasons behind their decisions. Still, this understanding only crystallized after extensive reflection, including countless hours of therapy, a robust support system, difficult life experiences, relationships that didn't work out, and a dedicated pursuit toward healing. During that period of reflection, I also read psychological journals and research studies, expanded my grasp on cultural differences, learned about the effects of childhood traumas, love languages, and attachment styles, and developed a greater understanding of how conditioned human behaviors come into play.

TOO MUCH AND NOT ENOUGH

Now let's examine how our familial relationships, patterns, and history can impact and shape our formative years.

As a child, I was not like the other kids. I could vividly recall specific moments from an early age—a skill I later recognized as a form of "photographic memory." My parents recognized my "gift," which led them to nurture and develop it throughout my upbringing.

This ability has remained with me into adulthood. One day, my family was gathered around the kitchen table, sipping tea, when I began recounting a memory of riding a bus in Russia. I described sitting at the back of the bus next to an older gentleman, my mother, and my grandmother. I detailed the conversations we'd had, the words exchanged with the older man, and how he'd gifted me a small toy. Even though I'd been barely two at the time, I could remember responding to him. As I narrated this memory, my mother began piecing it together. She was astonished that I remembered every detail of that day nearly three decades later, as she had long forgotten it.

I'm grateful to have had this skill during my formative years when I wasn't aware of how rare it was. It's given me an advantage in many situations, allowing me to retain and recall valuable information when others usually wouldn't be able to.

As I got older, I always wanted to improve myself and things around me and take on a leadership role. I, somehow, always felt as if I had so much to give and contribute. I just wanted to help and maybe make someone's life better. This feeling has always lived deep in the core of who I am. For example, in Grade 2, I organized a "garbage committee" in school. The kids would throw their garbage everywhere during recess, and something needed to be done to fix the problem. I organized a garbage pickup committee, recruited eleven people, got three teachers to approve the idea, acquired personal protective equipment, and created a pickup schedule.

Within two weeks, the playground was clean, the schedule was approved for weekly reoccurrence, and more kids wanted to participate. This awakened my entrepreneurial spirit, which, little did I know, would one day change my life.

However, I was always told I was both too much and not enough as a child. It was a paradox. I was considered too much because I was outspoken, hyper, had big ideas, took risks, and was not afraid to try new things or get out of my comfort zone, even if I was scared. For immigrant parents in a new country, this was hard to navigate, especially since I was always high energy.

I was a bit of a wild card for them, to be honest.

Simultaneously, I fell short in my parents' eyes because of my low elementary school grades, which they perceived as a reflection of their parenting. They believed that if their child did not achieve good grades or perform well academically, it indicated some failure on their part as parents.

However, my academic performance highly fluctuated. In the beginning, my teachers recognized my quick grasp of the school materials, and I skipped Grade 1 and was placed in an advanced program for Grade 2. However, as we will explore in Chapter 2, I was relocated and struggled, and my grades took a nosedive in Grades 3 to 5, shocking my parents.

What is important to note is that everyone has their own methods of absorbing information, and the traditional exams and academic systems do not cater to every type of learner. It was only later in life that I fully understood this, but during my younger years, I felt inadequate due to the mismatch between my learning style and the standardized testing format.

I know I am not the only one who has experienced this.

Neil Fleming's book *Teaching and Learning Styles: VARK Strategies*, which I read in high school, helped me understand my unique learning style.[5] Fleming identifies four primary preferred modes of learning:

> **Visual Learners** prefer to process information through visual aids such as charts, diagrams, maps, images, and graphs. They find it helpful to see information displayed clearly and in an organized way.

> **Auditory Learners** learn best through listening and hearing. They benefit from lectures, discussions, audiobooks, podcasts, and verbal explanations.

> **Reading/Writing Learners** prefer written materials. They absorb information by reading textbooks, notes, and assignments. They

also tend to take copious notes, as writing down the information helps them retain it better.

Kinesthetic Learners learn through physical engagement and hands-on experiences. They grasp concepts better when interacting with objects, participating in activities, and using their body to learn.[6]

In *Frames of Mind: The Theory of Multiple Intelligences*, Howard Gardner suggests additional learning styles.[7] He introduces the idea that intelligence comes in various forms:

Linguistic Intelligence is the ability to use language (one or multiple) effectively, such as through reading, writing, and verbal communication.

Logical-Mathematical Intelligence is the capacity for logical reasoning, problem-solving, and mathematical thinking.

Spatial Intelligence is the ability to perceive and manipulate visual-spatial information, such as in art, design, and navigation.

Musical Intelligence is the ability to understand, compose, and perform music and recognize melodic patterns and tones.

Bodily-Kinesthetic Intelligence is proficiency in physical activities, coordination, and body movement, often found in athletes, dancers, and performers.

Interpersonal Intelligence is the capacity to understand and relate well to others while displaying strong social and communication skills.

Intrapersonal Intelligence is the ability to understand oneself and one's emotions, motivations, and thoughts, leading to self-awareness and introspection.

Naturalistic Intelligence is sensitivity to and knowledge of the natural world, including a connection to nature, animals, and environmental phenomena.[8]

Gardner's theory suggests that everyone possesses a unique combination of these intelligences and has strengths and weaknesses within these frameworks.[9]

In retrospect, the reasons for my difficulties in school are clear. The school systems heavily emphasized auditory teachings, where teachers stood at the front of the room, verbally delivering lessons. Additionally, being removed from a familiar system and put into a foreign setting impacted my academic performance.

Hence, it was crucial for me to gain an understanding of my learning methods—so I did. According to Fleming's four learning modes, I am a visual and reading/writing learner. And according to Gardner, I have linguistic, bodily-kinesthetic, interpersonal, and intrapersonal intelligence.

I relate to the linguistic aspect the most. I'm a polyglot thanks to my parents' dedicated efforts. They taught me all the languages related to our family's culture, making me proficient in nearly four languages before age five.

I have a distinct memory of these practice sessions from a family video shot in my father's car. In the video, my father is asking me in Russian to recite numbers in various languages:

"Alright, Suzan, count in French."

"Un, deux, trois, quatre, cinq, six, sept, huit, neuf, dix."

"Bravo, Suzan! Now in Arabic," he says, beaming with pride.

"Wahid, itnan, talatah, arba'ah, hamsah, sittah, sab'ah, tamaniyah, tisah, ashara."

"Very good! And now in Russian."

"Odin, dvaaaaa . . ." I slow down.

"Come on, Suzan, quicker."

At this point, I start shouting at the top of my lungs. "TRI, CHETIRE, PIAT, SHEST, VOSEM, DEVIAT, DESIAT."

"Where is seven?" my father prompts.

I pause, whispering to myself, "Seven . . . ?" As soon as I realize my mistake, I resume with the same enthusiasm.

"SEM, VOSEM, DEVIAT, DESIAT."

"Bravo, Suzan!"

With repeated practice, engaging language games, and immersive experiences orchestrated and managed by my parents, especially my mother, I grasped the foundations of languages, making learning new ones feel like second nature. As I grew older, I became proficient in a few more to be able to relate to people from different cultures.

So, for my learning to be effective, I needed visual aids, written materials, multilingual social environments, and homework that I could review later. The schools I attended at an elementary level simply did not provide what I needed. But by learning what I needed, I was able to adjust. I accepted what had happened and acknowledged that this didn't make me a bad student; I had just lacked the resources to excel in school. When I finally found the resources that catered to my learning style, a transformation occurred in my academic journey. My grades dramatically improved, leading me to graduate high school and university with excellence.

I've shared this with you because schooling is a big part of our lives, particularly during childhood. Most of us spend at least thirteen years in formal education and many more if we pursue college, university, or various designations. Our grades often reflect our abilities on paper, influencing our opportunities in higher education institutions and determining the degrees we qualify for and the jobs available to us. However, it's never too late to recognize your unique learning style and take charge of your education, whether you're starting over or continuing your studies.

Each one of us possesses intelligence; it's simply a matter of discovering the approaches we need.[10]

I knew I had been misjudged, and I had the potential to excel academically. Determined to understand why I continued to struggle and get low grades, I sought solutions—a recurring theme you'll notice throughout this book.

From a very young age, I knew it was up to me to change my current situation. I looked for ways to overcome obstacles by myself because I knew that relying on others to fix things for me was not the answer or an option. I took responsibility for my circumstances and realized that if I had the ability to influence them, I should seize the opportunity.

While unexpected challenges can indeed arise, our actions and determination in the face of adversity can either make or break us, and it is within our power to rise above and chart our own path to success.

As a child, I remember constantly feeling as if I were walking on a tightrope, trying to balance who I was with who I was expected to be. It was challenging to be different. I never identified with other children my age and always thought I had to do more and be more. I often felt as though I possessed a deeper understanding, yet adults still saw me as a young child despite my ability to engage in discussions at their level.

That feeling continued during the week of 9/11, when teachers visited our classroom to gently ask if we were aware of what had happened. Little did they know that my family and I had been closely following the news in three languages and discussing the causes and repercussions of the incident. We had talked about the magnitude of the event and the potential geopolitical shifts it would bring about. I had just turned seven years old, but my parents never shielded my younger sister and me from information, especially concerning politics, the economy, and global affairs. Understanding and examining world events was a regular part of our lives.

When the teachers asked if anyone knew what had happened, I innocently raised my hand, and they invited me to the front of the class. With a piece of chalk, I began creating a visual representation, depicting the Twin Towers, the planes, and the people jumping to signify the gravity of the attack. I also discussed theories and the broader implications of the global security shift. At that moment, I was so passionate about sharing my knowledge that I didn't notice the silence in the room. When I turned around from the board, I saw horrified expressions on the teachers' faces, and some students were even in tears. I couldn't understand their reaction because, to me, this was the reality of the world we lived in.

The teachers sent a report to my parents, and I faced consequences at school for a few days. I was told not to continue sharing such information with other students, and I obediently followed their instructions. I was seven, after all.

Additionally, due to our family's Middle Eastern heritage, we faced further discrimination; it became so severe that my father completely stopped speaking with us in Arabic at home to ensure that we solely used languages that wouldn't bring us further adversity.

Regardless of the hardships, I knew I was destined to make some type of impact, even if I didn't know what it would be yet. That future impact—that enigmatic "it"—motivated me to move forward despite the limitations or beliefs imposed on me. I could never settle for "average." Deep within myself, I held the unwavering trust that my destiny was to experience life on a grand scale.

Now, as an adult, I can see how that "innocence" and "playfulness" that we have as children, where we believe that we are superheroes and can achieve and express anything that is on our minds, gets suppressed by many factors, and we lose that "spark" the older we get. I would have lost that childlike spark if I hadn't had that mysterious "it" filling me with purpose.

Parents, school systems, society, and even the corporate world try to mute or shut "it" down. We live in a world where being different and thinking and expressing ourselves outside the box is a risk, taboo, avoided, and discouraged. This is why so many people get to a certain age and regret that they didn't try to act on their ideas and succumbed to the rules imposed on them because of someone else's fears or limiting beliefs. Perhaps they went to university and got the "practical" or "safe" degree their parents wanted them to get instead of pursuing their creative passions, or they never started the business they dreamed of because of the uncertainty around entrepreneurship or the risk of failure behind it.

As I got into my late teens and early twenties, I realized I had been living my life based on my parents' agendas and adhering to societal expectations of me. Even though my parents encouraged me to get involved in extracurricular activities that stimulated me physically and mentally—well, as long as I maintained good grades, of course—they were strict. Even though my extracurricular activities delighted me, I lived a life that was not authentically mine. My parents' priorities had become my values, and I had somehow lost touch with my inner voice and genuine self.

It was not until I examined the patterns in my life that I began to understand the impact of those outside influences on my choices and actions. As they say, you can't unsee it once you've seen it.

THE WOUNDS OF CHILDHOOD

While we can acknowledge how our parents' upbringings and cultures impact our lives and decision-making processes, it's up to each of us to unlearn any negative patterns and behaviors that may have been passed down to us. As I mentioned at the beginning of the chapter, examining our origins is essential to uncovering their impact on us. My own unlearning process involved counseling and extensive reading on the subject, including *The Body Keeps the Score: Brain, Mind, and Body in the Healing of Trauma*, by Bessel van der Kolk.[11] This book gave me valuable insights and put a lot of things into perspective for me.

Childhood trauma can impact our physical, emotional, and mental health. We can avoid repeating the mistakes and experiences of our parents by taking responsibility for our growth and by improving our life circumstances, creating a healthier outlook for our children and future generations.[12]

Although the term "trauma" may evoke images of catastrophic events, it can also refer to seemingly minor experiences that end up greatly impacting a child's emotional, physical, and psychological well-being. These experiences can alter a child's brain development, leading to negative cognitive patterns that can persist into adulthood.[13]

It's not easy to talk about childhood trauma. It can be complicated and messy and bring up suppressed emotions; as a result, some self-help books avoid the topic altogether. But understanding the different types and their effects has been essential to my healing process.

If you've been through a harrowing experience, it's not enough to only acknowledge it; you must understand its impacts thoroughly to move forward. It might be uncomfortable initially, but I believe it's necessary to seek out this information if you haven't already. It may be the missing piece in your puzzle of growth. The forms of childhood trauma include the following:

> **Physical abuse**, which involves physical harm or injury caused by a caregiver.

> **Sexual abuse**, which involves any sexual act performed on a child.

Emotional abuse, which involves psychological harm inflicted by a caregiver, such as belittling, humiliating, or threatening a child.[14]

Neglect, which is when a caregiver fails to provide for a child's basic needs, such as food, shelter, and medical care.[15]

Children can also experience trauma from exposure to domestic violence, natural disasters, and accidents. These events can result in physical harm or emotional distress and can have long-lasting effects on a child's mental health.

Childhood traumas can cause feelings of abandonment, shame, guilt, and confusion and can affect a person's ability to form healthy relationships. As discussed in a document published by the National Center for Injury Prevention and Control, a caregiver can subject a child to psychological mistreatment in many ways, including "[b]ehaving in a manner that is harmful, potentially harmful, or insensitive to the child's developmental needs . . . [and b]ehaving in a manner that can potentially damage the child psychologically or emotionally."[16]

I have experienced the effects of unprocessed childhood events firsthand, though I want to emphasize that my experiences are not as extreme as some stories I have heard from people in my life and in the wider world. My intention in sharing my experiences is not to draw attention to myself but to share insights through storytelling. I aim to create a safe platform for exchanging information, to help you reflect on your own experiences.

As a child, I was programmed to believe that my worth was tied to my performance—that is, how well I completed tasks and obeyed authority figures. I had a daily routine of completing exercises written in a green laminated notebook my father gave me. The notebook covered several subjects, including mathematics, geography, writing, and cognitive memory activities. Doing well meant getting rewards, such as treats or pocket change, while poor performance led to discipline.

One day, I struggled with the math equations and got most of the answers wrong. My father took a bold red pen and marked my mistakes with big X's. He also left demeaning comments in the margins. Overwhelmed by a sense of failure, I felt tears stream down my cheeks and knew I would be isolated in my room until I mastered the exercises.

My father's words and actions hurt me, especially since that green book became a source of validation; when it was marked with red everywhere, I felt worthless. This particular aspect of my upbringing instilled a "reward system" mentality within me that affected my self-worth. For a long time, I believed that I had to gratify others to be liked and that any disapproval would lead to abandonment or punishment. This mindset conditioned me to become a people pleaser, which impacted my relationships as an adult. To this day, I am working on shedding that conditioned behavior.

Progress is rarely linear.

MOTHERS AND FATHERS

In her book *Adult Children of Emotionally Immature Parents: How to Heal from Distant, Rejecting, or Self-Involved Parents*, Dr. Lindsay Gibson explains that emotional neglect in childhood can cause challenges in forming healthy adult relationships and developing a strong sense of self.[17] She talks about how "emotional connection is a basic human need, regardless of gender . . . People who lacked emotional engagement in childhood, men and women alike, often can't believe that someone would want to have a relationship with them just because of who they are. They believe that if they want closeness, they must play a role that always puts the other person first."[18]

I believe that identifying specific experiences you had with each parent can bring about a better understanding of your perspective and beliefs, which influence you and the decisions you've made in your adult life—and that's where the mother and father wounds come in.

Dr. Gibson doesn't directly refer to the terms "mother wound" and "father wound" in her book, but the information she presents is similar to the thoughts and research I was exposed to, through different psychologists and professionals, regarding the concepts.

Differentiating between the mother wound and the father wound allows for a more nuanced understanding of an individual's emotional experiences. The relationship dynamics between a child and their mother are typically different from those between a child and their father. Each parent brings their own set of behaviors, communication styles, and emotional expressions, all of which can impact the child differently.

Mother wounds are inner injuries that stem from a lack of emotional nurturing, validation, or support from a mother figure. The causes of these wounds can include the following:

- Emotional or physical absence
- Verbal abuse, including belittling and body shaming
- Neglect
- Displaced aggression

These wounds can diminish a person's self-esteem, self-worth, and ability to form healthy relationships in adulthood. The effects of mother wounds can manifest in different ways, such as the following:

- Anxiety
- Depression
- Perfectionism
- Self-doubt
- People-pleasing
- Fear of abandonment

Over the years, I've learned about a few common signs that may indicate a mother wound.

> Having trouble establishing boundaries or advocating for oneself can stem from a mother who did not respect personal boundaries or was excessively controlling.
>
> Perfectionism and self-criticism can develop when a mother has unrealistic expectations or is overly critical. An individual may feel inadequate and as if they are unable to meet such high standards, leading to a persistent feeling of not measuring up.
>
> Fear of abandonment or rejection can result from a mother being emotionally unavailable, using silence as punishment, or being absent during childhood; these can create a fear of being left alone or losing the love and support of someone significant.
>
> Difficulty forming close relationships and trusting others can be related to receiving inconsistent love and support from a mother during childhood.

By contrast, father wounds refer to the emotional and psychological pain a person may experience due to their relationship or lack thereof with their father. Father wounds can manifest as feelings of the following:

- Rejection
- Abandonment
- Neglect

A person may have a father wound if they grew up with an absent, emotionally unavailable, abusive, or overly critical father. Here are some common signs of a father wound.

Challenges with trust, particularly toward male figures in positions of authority, can be a result of a father failing to keep promises or being disloyal.

Feelings of annoyance, anger, aggression, resentment, and bitterness toward a father figure might be transferred to other males in an individual's life.

There may be an inability to form and establish healthy relationships, particularly with males, due to insufficient positive role models.

Emotional numbness or detachment can be developed as a coping mechanism to protect the individual from ongoing emotional pain.

Healing from mother and father wounds and any other trauma can be challenging, but it is necessary for personal growth and well-being. Recognizing the signs and taking practical steps toward healing will catalyze your awakening and help you move to the next chapter of your life. It requires time, effort, and accountability. You will thank yourself later.

REFLECTIONS
ON TRAUMA HEALING

Here are some practical tips that helped me initiate my healing process. You may also find them helpful in your own journey.

As a first step, acknowledge and accept the experienced pain. This means facing the emotions and feelings that are buried deep inside.

Practice daily affirmations. You can use simple phrases such as "I am worthy," "I am content with who I am," and "I am enough." This practice can be a powerful self-support tool, as you should always try to be your biggest cheerleader.

Treat yourself with kindness during this process by remembering you are worthy of love and healing. Offer yourself the same love and compassion you would offer a close friend.

Remember that healing is not a journey you have to take alone. Having a support system of friends, family, and a therapist can help you feel heard, validated, and encouraged along the way.

Set healthy boundaries with your parent figure(s) if necessary to heal and protect yourself from further harm. This can include reducing the amount of time spent with a specific parent, restricting certain activities you engage in together, or declaring certain topics off-limits for discussion.

Make time for self-care activities that help you feel good and recharge your batteries. These can include exercise, meditation, journaling, or spending time in nature.

Keep in mind that these tips are broad suggestions—not all methods work for everyone. It's important to be creative and patient while finding the strategies that are best for you. Here are some alternate healing approaches you might consider:

Inner Child Work is a powerful tool for healing mother and father wounds. It involves connecting with the child within you and addressing the unmet needs and emotions from your childhood. This technique can help you develop a more compassionate and nurturing relationship with yourself.

Art Therapy helps individuals process and express their emotions in creative ways. It can be constructive and essential for those struggling to verbalize their feelings. Art therapy may involve painting, drawing, or sculpting.

Eye Movement Desensitization and Reprocessing is a type of psychotherapy used to treat trauma-related disorders. It involves reprocessing traumatic memories while simultaneously engaging in bilateral stimulation, such as eye movements or tapping.[19]

Body-Oriented Therapies focus on the relationship between the mind and the body. These therapies (such as somatic therapy) can help individuals release and process emotions stored in the body, which can manifest as tension or pain.

Breathwork is a type of therapy that involves controlled breathing exercises. It can reduce stress and anxiety and help individuals connect with their emotions.

If you are struggling, seeking professional help or reaching out to support groups can be incredibly beneficial, and thankfully, nowadays, there is less stigma attached to this. While the tips shared in this chapter are based on my personal experience, it is essential to note that they are not a substitute for professional advice or therapy.

It can be natural to feel overwhelmed as you confront unpleasant emotions and memories. Remember, it won't always be easy, but the rewards of personal growth are immeasurable. It takes work, bravery, and determination to face your struggles and fully understand yourself. The good news is that only you have the power to control your future and how you feel moving forward.

PEOPLE-PLEASING

As the firstborn of young immigrant parents, high expectations of me were inevitable—excellent performance was expected. I was constantly pushed to excel in every aspect of my life. Sometimes, I felt as though I had to be the perfect child, the shining trophy my parents could show off to the world. I didn't fully understand the impact this had on me at the time, but now, I see and know how it shaped my views on success and self-worth.

It's taken me some time to come to terms with the fact that my parents were doing the best they could with the tools they had, even if some of them did hurt me. Their upbringings and past experiences influenced how they showed love and support—even if, unfortunately, it wasn't always in the healthiest or most effective way. But I also understand that my parents were shaped by their parents, who didn't have the tools to show them what real love looked like. At that time, survival was the main goal, not love and compassion.

I now see and comprehend how my parents' upbringings and past ordeals influenced the way they raised me. They wanted to ensure I had the skills to succeed. And in many ways, they accomplished that. I became a machine with athletic abilities, fluency in multiple languages, a photographic memory, and a knack for geopolitics and business.

As a child, I didn't question my parents' methods. It wasn't until my late twenties that I realized how little I knew about boundaries and love. I had been raised in an environment where love was shown through toughness, discipline, and high expectations. Only when I learned about emotional intelligence did I realize that there was, in fact, another way.

What is emotional intelligence?

Daniel Goleman, in his book *Emotional Intelligence: Why It Can Matter More Than IQ*, defines emotional intelligence as the ability to recognize, understand, manage, and effectively use emotions in ourselves and with others.[20] He argues that emotional intelligence can be more crucial for success than traditional measures of intelligence (such as IQ), which I thought was very interesting. The book greatly emphasizes the importance of developing emotional competence through self-awareness, emotional regulation, and empathy.[21]

And so that is what I did: I showed empathy to myself, recognized the emotions that needed attention, and progressively initiated the appropriate changes in my life.

As we venture through the twists and turns of our journey, we might not always see how we unconsciously slip into the pattern of people-pleasing—a behavior where we prioritize others' needs and desires above our own. This inclination can be deeply rooted and often traces back to childhood.[22]

During childhood, we may have learned that we received approval and acceptance from others when we behaved in specific ways. Our parents or caregivers may have reinforced this by expressing love and affection only when we met a particular standard. Over time, we may have internalized this belief and come to see our worth as dependent on pleasing others and meeting their expectations—as I did with my green notebook.

Unfortunately, this pattern of behavior can persist into adulthood and lead to a lifelong habit of seeking validation and approval from others, even at the expense of our own needs and well-being. People-pleasing may also be a way to avoid conflict or negative feedback, as we fear that asserting our needs and boundaries will result in rejection or disapproval.

People pleasers often say yes to requests from others, even if the asks are unreasonable or not in their best interest. Taking advantage of this tendency can be a form of emotional mistreatment intended to punish or exert control over a people pleaser. For example, a family member or a friend may give a child the silent treatment to manipulate them into doing what they want, and the child may comply even though it is not a healthy or productive way of communicating. The silent treatment can lead to feelings of anxiety, depression, and helplessness. It can also cause the child who is being ignored to doubt themselves and their worth, resulting in damaged self-esteem.

In my household, any sign of unruliness was met with silence, leading me to become a people pleaser from a young age. I also developed hypervigilance, which meant I was acutely aware of every emotion and action in my immediate environment. I could discern the mood by paying attention to how those around me walked, talked, laughed, or even looked at me. I believe that, in my case, hypervigilance was a learned behavior rather than a result of childhood trauma, but it could be argued that it was a mix of both. All I knew at that time was that I needed to be in a constant state of alertness to gain approval and be validated. I couldn't be seen to make a mistake or burden someone with my perceived incompetence.

I was also hypervigilant outside of my home and earned the label of "teacher's pet" in late elementary and high school; I wanted every teacher to like me, so I took on extra activities, tried to perfectly understand the assignments to put myself in the best position to get the best grade, tutored others, and did whatever it took to be in their good graces. It brought me satisfaction and fulfillment to be recognized for my hard work, and that external validation made me feel seen and valued—which I didn't often feel at home.

People-pleasing tendencies can take many forms but are all rooted in the same underlying need for external validation and approval. Those who struggle with people-pleasing often have difficulty expressing their opinions or standing up for themselves. They may agree with others for the sake of agreeing, even when they don't believe what is said. People pleasers also avoid conflict because they fear upsetting others or being disliked. They may go to great lengths to avoid difficult conversations, even if it means sacrificing their needs and desires.

While seeking to please others might bring momentary relief, it can lead to resentment, burnout, and a lack of personal fulfillment in our relationships and lives. That's why it is crucial to recognize this pattern within ourselves.

Over time, I realized that it was okay if not everyone liked me. It was impossible to please everyone, and it wasn't my responsibility to make everyone like me. Understanding this and learning to set healthy boundaries allowed me to gradually unlearn these people-pleasing behaviors, one situation at a time. As I practiced self-restriction, I found healing and empowerment within myself.

NAVIGATING DIFFICULT INTERPERSONAL DYNAMICS

While I am not a psychologist or psychotherapist, my life experiences have motivated me to understand the complexities of human behaviors. Prolonged exposure to difficult and unexpected behaviors can cause irreparable damage to the psyche, and becoming aware of these behaviors lets us take steps to shield ourselves from harm, establish boundaries, and, perhaps more importantly, understand our impact on those around us.

By shedding light on these complex behaviors, we open the doors to healthier connections, greater self-awareness, and renewed inner strength. The book *Should I Stay or Should I Go: Surviving a Relationship with a Narcissist*, by Ramani Durvasula, Ph.D., explores emotional dynamics and personal growth; the book offers readers tools to navigate their emotions, assess their needs, and understand different behaviors, allowing them to make informed choices about their current relationships.[23]

Dr. Durvasula focuses a lot on the impacts of narcissism, and according to the *Diagnostic and Statistical Manual of Mental Disorders, Fifth Edition (DSM-5)*, which she references in *Should I Stay or Should I Go*, narcissistic personality disorder is a "pervasive pattern of grandiosity, need for admiration, and lack of empathy."[24]

As we've explored in this chapter, our personalities are formed early in life, and the parent-child relationship is a crucial factor in this. One theorist whose work I've found enlightening over the years is Otto Kernberg, whom Dr. Durvasula also mentions in her book. Kernberg proposed that "children who have unempathetic parents . . . will remain emotionally hungry throughout their lives and then develop their outer world instead of their inner world. Subsequently, they will overdevelop a skill set that the parents value (for example, appearance, academic achievement, athletic prowess, playing the violon) . . . [They] become masterful at compartmentalizing themselves, separating their world of achievement from everything else."[25]

Here are some of the tactics that narcissists employ.

Gaslighting is a form of psychological manipulation that aims to distort someone else's perception of reality, leaving them questioning their sanity and experiences. It is vital to recognize gaslighting as a weapon used to maintain control and undermine a person's sense of self.[26]

Manipulation involves influencing another's thoughts, emotions, and actions to serve their agenda. A manipulator will exploit someone's vulnerabilities using approaches such as guilt-tripping and emotional blackmail to achieve their desired outcomes.

Breadcrumbing is when they offer tantalizing glimpses of affection or attention only to withdraw abruptly, leaving the other person in a perpetual state of longing and uncertainty.[27]

Lying typically comes effortlessly to a narcissist, as it helps them to manipulate and control those around them. Their falsehoods can range from minor fabrications to elaborate deceit, all aimed at furthering their own interests and maintaining their disguise.[28]

Hoovering involves attempting to re-establish contact and suck another back into their web of influence and control, typically after a period of estrangement or separation.[29]

Exploiting the people in their lives to use them as apparatuses to fulfill their desires and aspirations. They lack genuine regard for others' well-being and value their presence only for the benefits they can provide.

We can also think of narcissists as "energy vampires" due to their draining nature. They feed off the emotional energy of those around them, leaving others depleted and emotionally exhausted.[30]

If you find yourself entangled in a relationship with a narcissist, seek help. Don't be hard on yourself; as Durvasula puts it, "Narcissism is basically the flame that draws in the moth."[31] There are resources available, such as therapists and support groups that specialize in dealing with the aftermath of narcissistic abuse. These avenues provide a safe space for healing and regaining control of your life.

BEGINNING TO HEAL

By recognizing the root causes of my struggles, I learned that emotional intelligence is not about controlling your feelings but about understanding and embracing them.

Truthfully, I learned what love and patience were when I got my dog, Mishka, a toy-sized Chihuahua and Pomeranian mix. She showed me what it means to have someone rely on you and how the weight of that responsibility cannot be taken lightly.

I came to this realization while potty training Mishka. I suspected she intentionally used the condo corners instead of the pee pad, and I struggled with this. Her failed attempts to use the pee pad aggressively irritated me—it was only later that I realized my irritation was similar to that of my parents when I did not comprehend something immediately.

One day, panic rushed through me as I observed her slowly moving toward the carpet under the coffee table. I ran toward her, and in my haste, I accidentally hit her chin on the corner of the table. She started bleeding, and I was filled with even more panic, hyperventilating, as I called the emergency vet.

In my distress, I found myself sitting in the bathtub with Mishka, covered in her blood, apologizing to her. Meanwhile, she was calmly licking my tear-stained face, offering comfort and solace; at that moment, something shifted. I stopped crying and looked at her injured four-month-old self. Despite my mistake, she was there, gently embracing me with her paws and providing unconditional kindness.

For those brief minutes, as she curled up on me, we connected on a deeper level. I realized that I had rushed her training. I hadn't given her the space and patience she needed to learn at her own pace.

I felt tremendous guilt.

After gathering my thoughts, I wrapped her up, changed out of my bloody clothes, and drove to the emergency vet. Throughout her recovery, Mishka cuddled with me, displaying affection and forgiveness despite the pain I had caused her.

This incident was a wake-up call for me. I had projected the negative behavior I had internalized onto Mishka, having not learned what it felt like to be understood or to have someone show me compassion and patience when I struggled or made a mistake. I know it might sound silly, but deep realizations can begin with simple moments like this.

Through her unwavering loyalty and unconditional love, Mishka opened my eyes to the true meaning of these virtues. She taught me to value patience and compassion in myself and others. Watching her grow, I realized how much I had missed out on as a child in that department and how much I craved this type of acceptance and understanding from those around me.

When I got my second dog, Tiapa, the experience was completely different. I could see that a healed approach is a game changer in relationships of any kind.

Like many others, my parents were burdened with generational wounds they could not heal from. We must remember that our parents are only human, and as we move forward, we should learn to forgive them and ourselves for the wounds that may never fully heal. We must exercise forgiveness for our own peace of mind.

While our formative years shape how we approach challenges in our lives, it's never too late to break free from those patterns and start living the lives we truly want—to gather enough *sisu* to break out of the nostalgia trap.

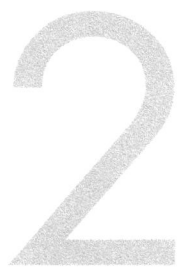

HIRAETH: ECHOES OF THE PAST

["Hiraeth": noun / 'hir, iTH/]
Deep longing for something, especially one's home.[1]

I WAS EIGHT when my parents left me in Russia with my grandmother, Babyshka.[2]

It happened unexpectedly, and I can still remember the sound of the train chugging away, growing fainter and fainter as I ran after it. Tears still stream down my face when I think about that moment.

We had been seated together—my mom, sister, Babyshka, and I—on the train, eager to head back home. But then Babyshka grabbed my hand and said it was time to get off. Confusion swept over me like a wave—why would I be leaving? Why was I staying in Russia while my sister and mother returned home?

Panic set in, and I couldn't hold back tears. My mother tried to comfort me, reminding me that we had discussed this before and that I was to stay in Russia for the summer to reinforce my native tongue and learn more about the culture. But as an eight-year-old, I had not fully felt the weight of that decision at the time.

I let Babyshka pull me out of the carriage, my heart heavy with distress. I stood there, helpless, watching as the train pulled away. Through the window, I saw my sister's tiny hand pressed against the glass as if to say goodbye. I felt so abandoned, so alone, wondering why I wasn't good enough to return home with my family.

The train platform was alive with the commotion of travelers, diesel fuel filled the air with its acrid smell, and trees swayed in the gentle breeze. It felt as if time stood still as I watched my family disappear from view. Tears blurred my vision as I ran after the train, begging it to stop. Babyshka ran after me, but she soon stopped and let me have my moment. But, as the train picked up its pace and I ran to the end of the tarmac, my heart pounded in my chest, and I could barely swallow or breathe as I saw the train disappear from my view.

And so began my abandonment issues, a wound that would haunt me for years to come.

In this chapter, I share the echoes of my past. It took me

twelve years of self-discovery to identify the root of the problem with my inner child: deep-seated abandonment.

Your experiences will differ from mine, but it's essential to understand and come to terms with your own past to heal and grow. We don't always realize that the small—and large—moments in our lives can affect our identities, emotions, and psyche. Discovering the root of my abandonment issues and finding forgiveness for myself and others allowed me to shed layers of anger and move forward with more peace and clarity.

BABYSHKA

What was initially intended to be a single summer stay was extended into a full academic year. And then another summer . . . And then another school year . . . One summer transformed into two years.

It was just Babyshka and me against the world for those two years. She became more than just a caregiver; she was my confidante, protector, and guiding light. She became my mother in every sense of the word. Let me take a moment to paint a picture of this remarkable woman.

Babyshka was the epitome of strength and resilience. She was a force to be reckoned with. She had soft blonde hair, piercing blue eyes, and an impeccable fashion sense. In her youth, she worked tirelessly as a train conductor, and she always put the needs of others before her own. She was the definition of kindness and selflessness.

Babyshka always prioritized my family and me; she visited us for months at a time when I was very young, and in later years, she even moved across the ocean just to be closer to us. She was more than just a grandmother; she was my savior, rock, and everything in between.

My grandfather, Babyshka's husband, passed away when I was only six. Although I have a few vague memories and a handful of old photographs and videos of him, I never truly knew him. The few stories that were shared with me painted a dark picture of a man with abusive tendencies. It's no wonder my mother and Babyshka rarely spoke of him; the impact of his behavior was likely felt long after he was gone. But in Babyshka, I still found a true example of love. She was a hardworking survivor who never let her past define her. Her kind heart and spectacular spirit were a constant source of inspiration, a reminder that there is always hope no matter how hard life may get.

Babyshka always found ways to make me feel special. One year, at Christmas, she adorned the Christmas tree with hidden toys; one was a doll with a stunning custom-made dress that she hid among the tinsel and ornaments. The fabric of the little handmade dress was a beautiful purple shade, complementing the doll's silky blonde hair, and I felt like a princess when I held it in my hands.

Our daily routine was always the same, yet it never grew old. Several days a week, even during the roughest winter days, she braved the snow and traveled four hours to take me to and from my gymnastics training. We would then rush home to watch the Brazilian soap opera *O Clone*, which started at 8:00 p.m.[3]

Babyshka had unconditional support to offer, even during tough times. We may have had little money for treats, but she always found ways to make life's simple pleasures memorable. For instance, Babyshka would search through the spoiling pomegranates in the bazaar and cut out the bad parts so I could enjoy the sweetest sections of my favorite fruit. She knew I loved olives, so she bought them for me instead of getting something for herself. Those small acts of kindness made me feel seen and loved.

Even my clothes were an expression of her love and care. Babyshka sewed all my costumes and outfits from scratch, taking great pride in ensuring I always looked my best. Whenever I wore one of her creations, I felt like a true fashionista. Her craftsmanship and attention to detail were unmatched.

Babyshka also had an unreal connection to nature. Her love for the outdoors was rooted in the belief that there was something divine and magical about the world, that it could heal and soothe the soul.

Before I came to live with her, she would take my sister and me on walks through the nearby meadows, and she would point out the different species of flowers, trees, and animals we encountered, encouraging us to stop and appreciate the beauty around us.

Our bike rides to our family garden in Russia are some of my fondest memories of Babyshka. She would pedal while I sat in the back, feeling every bump and jolt along the way. As we rode, she taught me to spot the common red cuckoo bird and the woodpecker. We always looked for them on our ride home.

I also loved watching her tend to her garden while I sat in an apple tree. She had a remarkable talent for making anything grow—from the tiniest seeds to the tallest trees. Watching her work was like witnessing a master at her craft. She moved with an effortless grace as if in perfect harmony with the earth. She would teach me how to plant a seed, nurture it, and care for it until it bloomed into a beautiful flower or a delicious vegetable. Her garden was a testament to her hard work and dedication, bringing joy and beauty to everyone who saw it. She often sat in her garden, taking in the fresh air, feeling the sun's warmth on her face and the soft grass beneath her feet. Her connection to nature was a constant reminder to be grateful for life's simple pleasures.

THE PAIN OF ABANDONMENT

Despite Babyshka's unwavering love, support, and efforts, I still felt the weight of abandonment on my shoulders during those two years in Russia.

I tried my best to fill the void. I realize now that I attempted in different ways to cope with the abandonment and emotional turmoil that I experienced. Still, at the time, it probably seemed like child's play outwardly. I was always overimaginative, mimicking the mannerisms of adults around me and the characters on my favorite TV shows and engaging in various creative pursuits.

I poured my soul into creating a world my family could be a part of, even if we were separated by distance and time. I started filming little videos to share with my loved ones once we were reunited, but simply documenting the mundane was not enough for me. I wanted to film something that would bring my family back to me, and that's when the Russian television show *Wait for Me* inspired me. The show revolved around the heart-warming pursuit of reuniting family members who had been separated by fate. The program followed its audience members as they searched for their long-lost loved ones with the help of skilled investigators and search teams, leading to tearful and joyous reunions that left viewers glued to their screens.[4]

Inspired by its format, I set out to capture my own search with the family's old camera and tapes in hand. I turned to my faithful audience of stuffed animals and poured my heart out. Each word was spoken with the hope that it would reach the ears of my "long-lost family" and ignite a spark of recognition that would lead them back to me. Looking through the lens, I imagined their faces once we were finally reunited. If it worked for the people on TV, it should work for me, too, right?

I found solace in more than just documenting my life in videos. I wrote my innermost thoughts and emotions in letters, sharing all the details of my experiences and longing for my family's embrace. My journal became my dearest companion, where I could safely express my deepest feelings, fears, and hopes without facing judgment or rejection.

Whenever I looked for new games to play, I imagined my sister's laughter and beaming smile when we could play together again. In quiet moments, I spoke to my family as if they were beside me, telling them about my day, sharing my dreams, and confessing my endless love for them.

I wrote to my parents, promising to study well so my dad would be proud of me, clean and be a good girl so my mom would be happy, and play hide-and-seek with my little sister so she would want her older sister back. I wrote many letters back then, and that was where my writing skills began to develop.

One day, however, many years later, my mother showed me some of the letters I had written, and I was surprised to see the anger I had poured into them. I don't even remember writing some of those angry letters. There was so much venom in them that it was hard to believe they had come from my young hand. But looking back on those letters, I could understand why I had written them. I had thought I wasn't good enough or loved. I was angry about being left alone and subconsciously made Babyshka the outlet for that anger. I lashed out at her in those letters, calling her names and saying that I didn't love her. But I didn't mean those words. Babyshka was my source of comfort and love in an uncertain and lonely world, but I lacked the emotional capacity and coping mechanisms to handle my complex emotions during that tumultuous period. I now know that writing those letters allowed me to express my emotions and work through my mayhem, even if what I wrote was not always kind.

It wasn't until I started receiving photos and updates from my family that the weight of their absence truly hit me. I had created a new world for myself with filming and writing, but no amount of imagination could fully shield me from the pain of seeing my family enjoying experiences I was not a part of.

The pictures they sent would come packaged with clothing and other little items. The photos were printed on glossy paper, showing my family camping in the woods, attending birthday parties, swimming in pools with slides, and staying at fancy hotels. Each photo was like a blow to my chest, a painful reminder of all I was missing out on.

To this day, one particular photo is engraved in my mind, and when I was reading this chapter to my sister during the editing stages, she stopped me and said, "The one with me in my swimsuit, eh?" Ha, she guessed right. It was a picture of my little sister standing on a plush hotel bed, her inflatable water wings wrapped around her arms, wearing a new swimsuit that I had never seen before. She looked so happy, so carefree. As I pored over the photos my family sent me, I couldn't help but feel jealousy and resentment. They were all smiles, enjoying their time at the pool and on their vacation. I only went to a pool once in Russia, a small, outdated one with my cousin. It was nothing compared to the grand, modern pools with colorful slides that my family frequented. The more I looked at those pictures, the more detached I felt from my family. Why didn't I deserve to be a part of those memories? Why was I left behind to only see them from afar?

My parents would call to speak with me on the phone, and at first, I was thrilled to hear their voices. But the conversations became increasingly strained; I preferred playing with the kids at the playground and stopped waiting for them to call. Time passed, and soon we had nothing in common, no shared experiences or memories to discuss.

ISOLATION AND BULLYING

The abandonment I felt in Russia was magnified by the bullying I experienced for being different, this time because I was a mixed-ethnic kid. I stood out with my appearance, last name, and unusual accent when speaking Russian.

It was challenging to make friends, and even the teachers seemed to treat me differently. When I put my hand up to participate, they didn't pick me, and I felt invisible. I always sat by myself at the last desk on the right in the classroom. Everyone else had someone to sit beside while I was in the back row alone. I thought everybody hated me, and my loneliness and isolation grew over time. The kids were getting verbal and physical with their taunting; I felt as if there would be no end.

The bullying and ostracization got so bad that Babyshka had to homeschool me for two semesters. I couldn't help but wonder where I had gone wrong and why I deserved such treatment. The experience devastated me as a child and rolled into my adult life without my realizing it.

Before I was homeschooled, school plays and concerts offered me an outlet. They marked every holiday season and allowed parents to watch their children perform. As a natural performer, I was in my element and would forget the daily bullying, even though the other kids called me a "show-off" for trying to express myself.

The teachers would try to fill the void of my parents' absence by giving me poems to recite and songs to sing about Babyshka. It was a kind gesture, but receiving "special treatment" because of my unorthodox circumstances only made me feel more isolated.

But there was one festive performance that I will never forget.

We were celebrating Mother's Day and had to learn a song from a cartoon called *Mom for Mammoth*.[5] It was a sweet story about a little mammoth who had been frozen for many years and was now on a journey to find his mother and ended up being adopted by elephants instead.

I felt like the lost baby mammoth; every word of the song we sang resonated with me. I knew that Babyshka was my elephant.

I stood on the stage among my classmates as they sang this song to their mothers, who beamed their big smiles and watched proudly from the audience, but I didn't have my mother there; I had only Babyshka. Although she became my mother figure, and I loved her dearly, it wasn't the same. I couldn't help but feel the emptiness in my heart. For most kids, it was a happy occasion, but for me, it was a reminder of what I didn't have.

I felt a lump forming in my throat, but I kept singing as I

moved to the back of the stage, trying to hide my tears. I was hoping that somehow my mother would hear me. And maybe, just maybe, she would come to find me.

GOING HOME?

The day had come, and I was finally reuniting with my family after what felt like an eternity. I felt a mixture of emotions—excitement, nervousness, and anxiety. I made my way through the airport, overwhelmed by the sea of people around me. Then, as the arrival gates opened, I saw my father, mother, and sister emerging, but as they approached me, it was like seeing strangers. My sister had grown up so much since I last saw her, and I didn't even recognize my parents. We hugged awkwardly and exchanged pleasantries, but it was clear that we were all struggling to connect.

We spent a few weeks in Russia and then flew back home. But where was home for me at that point?

Once we landed, we ordered a taxi to drop us off at "home." It was a house I'd never been to before; my family had moved there while I was in Russia. In the car, I looked out the window in confusion. None of it seemed familiar. It was a completely foreign place, and I didn't know anyone in the neighborhood. I was starting from scratch yet again.

I recall stepping out of the cab, and there on the balcony, a large dog stood barking. I couldn't contain my excitement and pointed at it, asking, "Wow! Do we have a dog?"

But my mother gently explained, "No, Suzan, that's the neighbor's dog. Our home is right beside theirs."

I felt a rush of anticipation as my family guided me to our front door. Inside, I received a quick tour of the house, which felt massive compared to the one-bedroom apartment in which I'd stayed with Babyshka for the past two years. My sister and mother led me to the room dedicated to my sister and me, but the only familiar sight in that room was the bunk beds we used to share in the old apartment. Everything else did not belong to me.

As I reveal my experiences in Russia and how they affected me, I also feel it's essential to share my sister's perspective from that time in our lives. She acknowledged that it couldn't have been easy for me, especially since I was "alone" in a foreign country while she remained with our parents, but she admitted that she was too young to fully understand why I had to leave.

A decade after I returned, we had an argument about my time in Russia. I don't recall exactly how it started, but it was inevitable that the emotions would resurface. With tears, she said, "Do you think it was easy for me? My older sister was just taken away from me. One day, you were there; the next, you were gone for a long time. I was sad, and I wanted you with me. You were my protector, and you always had my back." She essentially had to adapt to doing things alone without her sister by her side.

The entire time I was gone, my sister still slept in the bottom bunk of the bunk beds we'd shared, and the top bunk, where I used to sleep, remained empty. We shared a room for almost fifteen years, and those bunk beds were the one constant in our lives. We used to have a little tradition where we wished each other good night every evening, and my sister confessed that during my absence, she continued this tradition every night before going to sleep. She told me, "I would always say, 'Good night, Suzan' to wish you a good sleep, even though I knew you weren't there to respond to me." When she shared that with me, we both started crying and hugged tightly. It was a moment of shared understanding and healing between us.

Upon returning from Russia, I had to once again adapt to a new environment. Even simple things such as operating the sink in the bathroom seemed like a challenge. The sink had one of those handles that you had to lift up and then move left or right for hot or cold water; I had only ever been exposed to knob-style sinks before, so I didn't know how to use this one. As I stood there trying to get the tap water running, awkwardly navigating the handle left and right without actually lifting it, I felt embarrassed that I didn't know how to do something so basic. It was the same with everyday products such as shampoo and conditioner. I had never heard of conditioner before and didn't know how to use it, so I left it in my hair. When my mother was trying to dry my hair with a towel, she asked me why it was so sticky. I innocently responded that I thought I had to leave it in as I'd never used it before. At that point, I felt self-conscious because I was ten years old, but it felt as if I was learning to walk all over again.

At school, I thought I would finally have a chance to start fresh. But to my dismay, the same pattern of bullying repeated. I was once again different from the other kids, making me an easy target. They picked on me for my accent, clothing, and candid nature.

Like in Russia, I didn't understand why I was so unlovable and why kids and adults easily dismissed me. And to make the situation worse, I didn't receive the support and reassurance I needed at home. Instead, I was blamed for the bullying and was told that I must be doing something to provoke it. Once again, I was left to fend for myself.

The only solace I found was in the company of the teachers, especially in high school. I spent all my free time in the teachers' lounges chatting with them. It was a way to escape the isolation and bullying that seemed to follow me everywhere.

Even though I was reunited with my family, it didn't feel like home. But I adapted, and eventually, I found my place. I learned that home isn't just a place; it's a feeling. I created a *home* within myself. When home is within you, it doesn't matter where you are physically.

LETTING GO OF ANGER

I was on a mission to get closure when I returned to Russia twelve years after I left. I held a grudge against my elementary schoolteacher this entire time. I visited the school and found out she was still working there. I was given her phone number, and I called her. As soon as she heard my voice, she said, "Suzanna?" I couldn't believe she remembered my voice and my name after so long, and I asked her if I could see her the next day. She enthusiastically agreed.

Within the first few minutes of seeing her, I blurted, "I have been upset with you for over a decade." She seemed confused to hear this. To my surprise, she told me that she always thought I was a special kid and that she remembered me as one of the most unique students she'd taught in her career. Once I heard that, I couldn't hold back; I began venting about all the bullying, the pain I felt while sitting at the back of the classroom, the feeling that all the teachers, including her, were against me, and that I wished someone had protected me during those times. She listened patiently without interrupting until I had let it all out.

"Oy Suzanna," she began, heaving a massive sigh, "it's unfortunate that this is how you remember your time here. Yes, the kids were not kind to you because you were not like them. They had never encountered someone from your background, and even though I could see how challenging it was for you to adapt to studying different subjects in Russian—you were a special kid."

Hearing about the bullying from her perspective was surreal, but her words were a relief. Finally, someone had acknowledged my experience rather than blaming me for how others treated me.

She went on. "You must understand that the other kids were jealous, and it had nothing to do with you being unlovable or not enough. I purposefully sat you at the back of the classroom to shield you from the nastiness they were putting you through.

Sometimes, I didn't pick you to prevent their envy from escalating further. You were special, and they knew it. They wanted to be like you but couldn't, so they lashed out in retaliation."

"As for the teachers," she continued, "it was a different story. We pushed you harder because we saw your academic potential. You were bright, and I spent countless hours with you, helping you learn to read and write according to the curriculum so you could catch up. Your mother and I even exchanged emails to ensure you received the appropriate French tutoring to retain the language. I am sorry again that you felt this way all those years. Someone should have explained this to you. I hope you understand everything better now as an adult. It was jealousy, not a reflection of you."

She's right. Someone should have taken the time to explain it to me. Instead, I was always just blamed for the poor treatment and told I deserved it because of who and how I was. Over the years, this perception caused me so much emotional damage that I became a serial people pleaser to cope and avoid more confrontations. I felt as if I needed to overcompensate in every aspect of my life to feel loved, which only worsened my perception of things.

I stared at my former teacher silently for a full minute, taking in her expression and body language. It was a significant moment in my life, and I wanted to preserve every detail.

I got my closure.

After that conversation, I stormed off to see my mother, who was with Babyshka, at the family apartment. I told her everything that my teacher had told me. I was raging, out of control, shouting, letting out the anger that had festered inside me for years. All it would have taken was for her, or anyone, to tell me that it wasn't me, that I was loved, and to show me support and kindness when I felt defeated. That would have prevented the daily turmoil and doubt I felt practically the entire time I was in Russia and in school when I came back.

That day, my inner child began to heal.

REFLECTIONS
ON SEEKING CLOSURE

If you are prepared to seek closure, here are some steps you can take.

- Begin by acknowledging and accepting your emotions, allowing yourself to feel them without judgment.
- Reflect on the events and people who have affected you, recognizing their impact on your life.
- Practice self-compassion and forgiveness toward yourself and others involved.
- Engage in reflection while journaling to gain insights. Writing your thoughts can help release a mental load. Once you see everything on paper, you can reflect more easily.
- Seek support from trusted friends, family, and a therapist, as talking about your experiences can be incredibly cathartic.
- Set healthy boundaries to protect yourself from further triggers and prioritize your well-being.

Remember, closure is a gradual process, and starting with small steps at your own pace is okay.

Other people might not be able to provide you with the necessary closure. Even though it could be very helpful at times, it isn't their responsibility. Some are just not capable. Therefore, finding closure for *yourself* on your own terms is essential, as it allows you to make peace with past experiences and emotions. It empowers you to let go of unresolved feelings and move forward with renewed strength and clarity. Closure ultimately brings a sense of finality and completeness, freeing you from the weight of unfinished business.

Russia was where a lot of my mental growth occurred, and despite the many challenges, I shared some truly magical moments with Babyshka that would never have happened had I not been there with her. I am grateful for the incredible woman she was for me during those years and throughout my life. Her unconditional love saved me, shaping the person I am today.

I realize how fortunate I was to have those experiences with Babyshka because they gave me a deep appreciation for different cultures and ways of life. My time with Babyshka stands out as the highlights of my childhood; with her, I had a chance to experience a completely different life from that of my peers in the West.

The downside was that my abandonment issues had created a hyper-independent perfectionist who didn't know how to ask for help. These were defense mechanisms that helped me survive, but through healing, I began letting go of these patterns and rewired my ideologies and behaviors.

It was up to me to evaluate and understand the echoes of my past so I could move forward and create the life I truly desired.

3

~~STEADFAST:~~ UNWAVERING AMID CHANGE

["Steadfast": adjective / 'sted,fast/]
Firm in belief, determination, or adherence: LOYAL.[1]

MY EARLY CHILDHOOD HOME was filled with the sound of music, the rhythmic thump of our dancing feet, and traditional family moments that we cherished. Our living room was often a stage, and we took turns as performers. My parents never let the challenges they faced define our home. Instead, they made it a sanctuary where we could always find joy and solace in creative expression.

Some memories have burrowed deep inside my consciousness. One of my favorites is captured on a home video from when I was six; my younger sister was only two. In her usual fashion, my mother dressed us in adorable little dresses and set up an improvised dance party. She played a popular album by Tarkan, a Turkish artist then at the height of his popularity, which my dad had bought for me despite our limited funds. The music filled the room, and my sister and I danced while our mother recorded us on the family video camera.

When I read this chapter to my father, a smile lit up his face. We paused, and I couldn't help but ask him about the reason for his wide grin.

"Do you know how much the album cost?" he asked, still smiling.

"Um, around $15.00 or $20.00," I replied.

"No, it was around $50.00. That's equivalent to ten hours of work at $5.00 per hour. But you really wanted it, and it brought me joy to get it for you. What's funny is that I had to go to a specific store: HVM, HRA . . ." He trailed off as he tried to remember.

I interrupted. "HMV!"

He continued with a chuckle. "Yes, yes, HMV. Trying to find that cassette for you turned into quite an adventure, to say the least."

We both laughed, and I resumed reading.

I am indebted to my parents for filming every moment of our lives from birth, ensuring we had a tangible link to our past as we grew up. During my time in Russia, it was those "documenting" behaviors that I imitated to cope with my loneliness. It made me feel as though I belonged and was making a meaningful contribution to our family's memoir.

I continued this tradition even in my early twenties, spending seven months digitizing all our videotapes and creating a four-hour movie that encapsulated twenty-five years of my family's life, from my parents' wedding videos to our experiences in adulthood. Documenting and safeguarding memories has become an integral part of my identity.

As I watch the videos now, I can't help but be struck by how young and lighthearted my mother appeared. My mother was a professional dancer in Russia, an artist who knew how to move with grace and precision, and she passed on that love of dance to her children. Her dedication to dance was just one aspect of her character that I admired. She did well with whatever she put her mind to, whether it was academics, organizing and planning, creative pursuits, or anything in between. She was a perfectionist, and that trait rubbed off on me.

At times, I still feel the soft carpet beneath my feet, see the sunlight pouring in through the window like a spotlight, and hear my mother's laughter as she twirled around the room with her flowy skirt and long brown hair. My mother was a natural performer, her body expressing what words could not, especially when our father was away studying and working to provide for us.

I occasionally watch those videos to humble myself and remember that those experiences shaped who my parents are today. It's difficult not to empathize with all they endured during those years. They were only human, and they did their best—after all, they're also experiencing and navigating life for the first time too.

Those early years of dancing and self-expression contributed significantly to who I am, and my parents saw that and took the time to nurture it, crafting unique skill sets that I would draw from for years to come.

In this chapter, I'll dive into the many early experiences and achievements that brought valuable lessons into my life. We all have stories of hope and despair in our pasts, and I'm no different.

OLYMPIC DREAMS

As I mentioned in Chapter 1, I had an enormous amount of energy as a child. I was always eager to run, jump, and climb any object within reach. My parents once told me our neighbors commented on my abilities and jokingly suggested I join the circus. They were astonished when they saw me flip four feet off the ground from the monkey bars at only two years old.

My parents signed me up for rhythmic gymnastics before I turned five, and my existence began to revolve around those energy-draining training sessions. This sport was my calling. It was a haven where I could depend solely on my abilities and no one could affect the outcome of my actions except me. My goal was clear: to rise to the ranks of a professional athlete and someday compete in the Olympics.

I was not gifted with the innate agility of a gymnast, like some of my peers who were born with double-jointed knees or backs. I possessed something else: the conviction that I could achieve anything I set my mind to. But this also meant I had to work twice as hard to refine the skills that came effortlessly to others.

I never let that discourage me, but unfortunately, many individuals might have been. I've seen it happen around me multiple times. Most people tend to confine themselves within self-imposed limitations, convinced they lack the qualifications, experience, or talent for a particular pursuit, as if they don't fit neatly into a predefined "box." But why are we so obediently adhering to these restrictive boundaries imposed on us?

Only when we recognize that we control our outcomes, regardless of our circumstances, can we unleash the full potential of our abilities. I believe in at least trying to challenge the status quo for our own sake.

I knew that the result I wanted depended solely on my willpower—a fact that I found scary but also comforting. It meant that I was responsible for my successes and defeats. What I sowed was what I would reap.

One day at training, we were learning how to do standing bridges. This required us to raise our arms and arch our backs while keeping our hands in line to land gracefully on them upside down. Misplace your hands and you could wind up on your head or back.

I can't count how many times I fell. If I hurt myself, it was my fault—no one else was to blame. So, I executed that move repeatedly until I mastered it. I learned to trust myself despite the fear and uncertainty I felt.

I approached every other gymnastics skill with that mentality for the next three years.

After years of dedicated practice, I was told by my coach that I had been selected to train for the Provincials. The exhilaration I felt was indescribable. I had taken one giant leap closer to realizing my goal.

But alas, destiny had other plans in store for me, and my path to glory would be far from linear. The sudden relocation to Russia disrupted that goal and dream.

WANTING TO SOAR

In Russia, my primary goal was to continue with rhythmic gymnastics. However, the nearest school that offered this discipline was two hours away each way. Despite the distance, Babyshka came through, and we would spend four hours on the road almost every day, even in the cold, grueling Russian winters, to ensure that I could keep up my athletic momentum. We did that for nearly six months until one day at school, something unexpected happened that would redirect my path again.

The school had arranged a surprise for us on the Russian "day of sport": a circus performance. I remember watching in awe, completely mesmerized by the acrobatic feats. It was a whole new world of physicality and artistry, and it was incredible to see it up close. My curiosity was immediately piqued, and I knew I had to be a part of it.

I asked to put gymnastics on hold and to enroll in the circus and acrobatics school instead. It wasn't an easy choice, but the proximity of the school and the temptation of learning new skills won Babyshka and me over. And just like that, my life took another 180-degree turn. I was no longer a rhythmic gymnast; I was now a circus trainee.

By the age of nine, I had accumulated a vast reservoir of skills in acrobatics, and I was deeply in tune with my physical abilities. Two renowned coaches who possessed charismatic yet authoritarian personalities were devoted to instilling the virtues of discipline and focus in me.

In the circus world, before being assigned to a specific craft, we had to grasp the fundamentals of each discipline. We practiced hand and feet acrobatics, partner acrobatics, juggling, knife handling and throwing, the art of falling, aerialism, and other core proficiencies.

I loved every discipline and wanted to immerse myself in them all. However, due to my achievements in rhythmic gymnastics, one of the coaches—the youthful one who always believed in putting on a show—cultivated my Hula-Hooping talents. However, I was a little bitter about his choice of craft for me since I yearned to soar through the air as an aerialist. I advocated for it relentlessly, only to be told: "Suzanna, to truly excel, you must focus on one pursuit, not juggle three to five at a time." How ironic to be advised against juggling at the circus! Despite my wishes, I was still assigned the Hula-Hoop act and was allowed to indulge in aerial endeavors only between practices.

My coach's words still echo in my mind. There's a grain of truth in them cautioning against becoming a mere jack-of-all-trades. Yes, a specialization certainly has advantages, but being open to possibilities is equally valuable. In hindsight, I believe my coach's insistence was an attempt to enforce his own limiting principles on me; perhaps it was a burden enforced on him in the past. It showed me that even those with the greatest intentions can inadvertently suppress one's growth.

Working with Hula-Hoops was difficult, especially with older equipment. Instead of the sleek and lightweight plastic hoops available today, we used clunky metal ones. I wish you could hear their loud noises each time they fell against the wood floor. Those metal hoops also left an array of ugly bruises on my knees, ribs, and wrists. I had a rainbow of purple marks for most of my circus days. Sometimes, I couldn't even touch them without shedding a few tears. Yet, I wore them with pride, knowing that they represented a sacrifice for the art that set my soul on fire.

My circus detour ended up teaching me to dream even further, defy the odds, and embrace the full extent of my potential. Now, I had the confidence to explore, test my limits, and unlock the performer that had always resided within me. In the circus, I discovered that limits exist only to be shattered, and I gained even stronger discipline and focus.

I heard people say a few times, "It'll happen if it's meant to be." But why do we make the mistake of naively assuming that we can leave everything to chance? In reality, the trajectory of your life is in your hands. I learned this firsthand in my pursuit to be taken seriously as an aerialist. While my peers took breaks from their grueling sessions, I used every moment to practice. I ended up proving my worth and earned the right to fly. But that outcome was only possible through relentless determination and self-imposed training. I refused to accept no as an answer. Instead, I worked twice as hard to prove my competence and passion for the craft. Sometimes, all it takes is doing things many are unwilling to do.

Once you realize that this attitude is applicable beyond the realms of the circus, you can fly on your own terms. We live in a globalized world that thrives on cutthroat competition, after all. So, own your skills and find ways to set yourself apart in whichever industry you are in.

Those who understand the power of discipline, establish routines, and hold themselves accountable will surge ahead. The stark truth is that it's solely up to *you* to instill and incorporate that mindset and practice into your life.

REFLECTIONS
ON ACQUIRING SKILLS

To help you stand out from the crowd, here are some tips for focusing on personal and professional development while acquiring specific skills and knowledge.

- Make a list to understand your strengths, weaknesses, values, and passions. This introspection will help you align your pursuits with your identity.
- Become a lifelong learner, stay curious, and be open to new knowledge and ideas. Seek formal and informal education, attend workshops, read books, and take online courses to expand your expertise.
- Identify areas that interest you and acquire specialized skills relevant to your field. You can become an expert in a particular domain or diversify your skills until one genuinely stands out.
- In a rapidly changing world, be adaptable and flexible. Embrace new technologies and trends and be willing to pivot when necessary. Being able to adapt like a chameleon is a fantastic skill to have.

- Sharpen your communication skills, both verbal and written. Learning an additional language can open new doors and enhance cultural awareness.
- Build a strong professional network. When possible, attend events, conferences, and industry gatherings to connect with like-minded individuals and potential mentors.
- Don't fear failure; see it as an opportunity instead. Cultivate resilience to bounce back from setbacks. Failure is natural when you start stepping out of your comfort zone.
- Establish a unique and authentic brand that represents your values, differentiators, and what you bring to the table. Answer the question "Why you?"
- Most importantly, follow your passion and align your career choices with what truly ignites your soul.

Remember that differentiation is not about being completely different from everyone else; it's about emphasizing your unique qualities, strengths, and contributions. You can set yourself apart and thrive in a competitive world by continually improving yourself and offering value in your chosen sphere.

THE QUEEN'S GAMBIT

Chess was another passion I developed in Russia. I can't recall exactly how I got into the game or learned the rules, but it felt like a cultural tradition I had to embrace, and I excelled quickly. I read chess books, meticulously transcribed games, and started participating in competitions. I even placed in a few regional competitions in Russia. Upon returning home, I proudly led my high school's team as its first female chess team captain.

Chess taught me the art of strategy, honing my ability to

think three moves ahead, interpret my opponents' body language, and contemplate best- and worst-case scenarios within seconds. My hypervigilance proved advantageous here, allowing me to anticipate the opponent's next move by carefully observing their every action, where their gaze fell, and their reactions to my moves. The world around me seemed to freeze during each game, making me feel as if I were immersed in a psychological drama like *The Queen's Gambit*.[2]

All the experiences and skills I accumulated in my youth taught me that self-reliance fosters trust in one's ability to defy the phantom of failure. Failure became an enigma in my life; I acknowledged that I controlled its influence on me. But this fortitude did not materialize overnight; I spent years cultivating it long before I confronted the myriad challenges of adulthood.

Every experience, triumph, and setback we have encountered has led us to this exact moment. The beauty of it all is that we are never starting from zero; we carry within us the foundations and experiences that have shaped us thus far in our journeys.

In my life, I have met many people haunted by the paralyzing fear of failure that shackled their dreams and condemned them to a life of complacency. Too often, individuals surrender to the siren call of comfort, relinquishing their aspirations in favor of a sedated existence dictated by their circumstances.

However, even those brave enough to take risks and achieve what they want can also be secretly afraid of success. When the spotlight shines, victory is theirs, and a new set of responsibilities and pressures comes crashing in. It's like a different game they didn't know they were playing, and they're now afraid to lose.

Learning to trust ourselves and our instincts, even in the face of fear, is among the most imperative and valuable skills we can develop. Self-belief is a strong force that empowers us to navigate the labyrinthian path before us, allowing us to defy the odds and surpass the limited life we once settled for.

REFLECTIONS
ON SELF-DISCOVERY

Knowledge of yourself, your values, and the emotions you attach to significant aspects of your life will help you achieve your goals. To help identify the obstacles that could hinder you in pursuing your desired path, I've created a list of self-reflection topics for you.

- Assess where you currently are in life, objectively examining your circumstances, achievements, and challenges.
- Ask yourself, where do you aspire to be in six months, one year, and three years. Set tangible targets to strive for. Try to divide them into short- and long-term goals.
- Identify and list the personal, family, and traditional values that guide your decision-making and define your character.
- Recognize the skills you already possess or want to acquire, such as languages, academic competencies, street smarts, and life experiences.
- Evaluate your life's positive and negative influences, including relationships with colleagues, friends, partners, and family members.
- Take stock of your responsibilities, such as financial obligations. Assess your current financial standing and consider any improvements you wish to make, such as increasing savings, paying off some debt, or making significant purchases.
- Reflect on the state of your well-being, both mentally and physically, identifying areas where attention may be beneficial.

- Pinpoint specific areas of your life where you desire growth and development, and consider any additional factors that hold importance to you.

Once you've gained some clarity through personal reflection, it's time to transform your aspirations into a concrete action plan.

- Take time to network to surround yourself with like-minded individuals who share your goals and can support you or provide additional resources.
- Recognize your current behaviors and routines that may impede your growth and create strategies to overcome them.
- Break down your goals into manageable steps, creating a road map for their realization. Ensure each step is actionable and measurable, allowing you to track your progress and celebrate your milestones.

You can realize your true potential only once you embrace the trials and triumphs of self-discovery. Trust yourself, follow your instincts, and embrace possibilities when faced with uncertainty.

My time in the circus and playing chess instilled a mindset of discipline in me. Those experiences marked my entry into a life packed with professional discoveries, achievements, and challenges. Sometimes, I wonder what became of the artists and coaches I spent months training and sharing blood and sweat with in our quest to learn new skills. Did they learn the same life lessons I did? What did they discover about themselves along the way?

COMING HOME TO GYMNASTICS

When I returned to the place I called "home," I enrolled in a small rhythmic gymnastics school. However, I was not the same gymnast I'd been before leaving for Russia; I was now a gymnast with a multifaceted skill set, unafraid of the grueling labor required to succeed. And because of that, I was immediately placed to compete on a Provincial level. It was the completion of a perfect circle, a return to the very point where I had left off.

However, I quickly discovered that balancing academic commitments and athletic pursuits can be delicate. I had to attend school from 8:00 am to 3:30 pm; after school, I dedicated an hour to doing homework, trained from 5:00 pm to 9:00 pm, and then spent an additional three hours on other academic assignments. This carefully crafted schedule helped me excel academically while allowing for the pursuit of my athletic passions. This lifestyle, naturally, gave me little room to develop a social life. What soothed my longing for "normal" social interactions was meeting my best friend, Sarah, at gymnastics. We did everything together, within and outside our craft, and our parents even arranged a carpool schedule for us.

Becoming friends wasn't something we initially had in mind—in the beginning, we didn't even particularly like each other. Sarah was somewhat reserved, while I was a bit of a firecracker. However, we lived within walking distance of each other, so our parents organized the carpool to streamline their schedules. And so it began, with me sitting in her car with the limited grasp of English I had at the time, making proper interaction a challenge, and yet we had to share the car several times a week.

The culture shock Sarah experienced with my family was an added humorous twist to our friendship. On one occasion, she hopped out of my family's car and said, "Suzanna, it's surreal. You and your mother converse in Russian, then you swiftly switch to speaking French with your sister, and all the while, there's Arabic or Russian music playing in the background. I sat there, thinking, 'What have I signed up for, and where am I?' You guys are quite the whirlwind experience." But Sarah and I forged a stronger bond week by week, cultivating a friendship that would last a lifetime.

As my life unfolded, Sarah stood steadfast by my side, and her presence and support would play a central role in my story. Together, we braved the turbulence of adolescence, and our shared aspirations and moments of joy were the fabric that wove our destinies together.

Shall we continue? I took a momentary detour in the narrative.

I climbed the gymnastics ranks, within a few years, I was allowed to compete at a Junior National level. As I ventured into national and international arenas, I became even more determined to become an Olympian. At that point, every aspect of my life was aligned to pave the way for this monumental achievement.

In all these aspirations, a prominent figure stood by my side —my mother. She was my rock, providing support and guidance throughout those formative years. With an unshakable belief in my abilities, she fueled my confidence and nurtured my athletic growth. Our shared passion for gymnastics became the cornerstone of our bond.

Down to the detailed stitching of my costumes, my mother's influence impacted every component of my gymnastics ambitions. She assumed the roles of chauffeur, companion, music editor, videographer, and mentor, ensuring I never missed a training session or competition. Hours upon hours were spent together in the gym as she coached me on artistry after she'd already put in a full day at work. This is where her background in dance found a new purpose. Drawing from her wealth of experience, she guided me in expressing myself through fluid movements, collaborating with my coaches to select the perfect music, helping choreograph my routines, and introducing innovative movements to captivate judges and the audience.

My mother's commitment shone brightly in this partnership. Together, we navigated the rough waters of training and competition, united by a shared vision. I knew that was my mother's way of expressing her love, and it played a pivotal role in shaping the athlete I became.

ON DECK

One day, my coach received a letter inviting me to a summer camp, an exclusive opportunity to train at an Olympic level and then potentially join a group that would compete on the grandest stage—the 2012 Summer Olympics in London, England. The realization struck me like lightning: I had been pre-selected for the Olympics.

From that moment forward, every aspect of my training was laser-focused on preparing for that summer camp. Flexibility became an obsession, skills were refined, apparatus techniques were sharpened, and ballet became essential. It was a relentless pursuit of perfection, a tangible manifestation of my dream inching closer to reality.

But despite all my eagerness, I knew I did not possess the same ability level as some of the more seasoned gymnasts. Many of my peers were older and had more experience, and I had one other added difficulty: I was a lefty in a predominantly right-legged world. This meant I executed tricks and techniques differently, making synchronizing movements in a group setting inherently more challenging.

I persevered, determined to prove that my commitment could overcome any perceived disadvantage. And so I advanced to the next stage of training at the summer camp—an exclusive milestone. My dream of Olympic glory seemed within reach.

During my training, I learned the "on-deck mentality." A gymnast is on deck while waiting for their turn when another is competing. So when I was on deck, I had two options: stand there observing my competitor, or tune out my surroundings and try to get into my focus zone. Being on deck often brought a mix of nervousness and anxiety, sometimes to the point of nausea. There were moments when I would even momentarily forget my routine due to this hidden panic. On the outside, I appeared calm, but inside, I was a storm.

However, something would always change when my name was announced and I stepped onto the carpet. It felt as if I put on noise-canceling headphones and became fully activated, like a robot. The nervousness vanished, and I became oblivious to the sounds of applause or the announcer introducing the next gymnast on deck. I would enter my own world, assuming the position and ready to complete the mission I trained for.

Mastering the ability to focus and perform despite fear and nerves was one of the biggest strengths I acquired as a gymnast. The arena, the crowd's gaze, and the weight of expectations can often trigger overwhelming feelings; yet, in these moments of heightened pressure, I honed an ability to harness my fears and channel them into energy that enhanced rather than hindered my performance.

REFLECTIONS
ON RESILIENCE

Resilience in the face of fear and nerves is rooted in psychological and practical strategies. These are some of the techniques I used to cultivate this skill as an athlete that can potentially apply in different areas of your journey.

- Visualizing successful routines and imagining yourself confidently navigating the competition enhances focus when nerves surge.

- Consistent and thorough training is vital. When routines and skills become second nature, they act as a stabilizing anchor.
- Mindful breathing techniques can help you manage nerves. Deep, controlled breaths help regulate the body's stress response and clear the mind for focused execution.
- Address the physical symptoms of fear—such as a racing heart and trembling limbs. Exercises such as grounding techniques can involve sensory experiences that engage the five senses (sight, sound, touch, taste, and smell) to redirect attention away from distressing thoughts or feelings.
- Reframing fear as a natural response to a challenging situation helps normalize the experience.
- Record and then analyze each performance, regardless of the outcome. Learning from both successes and setbacks can refine your resilience-building process, in turn adjusting how you train.

Gaining insight into my responses while building and learning the benefits of resilience has enabled me to pursue any endeavor with motivation and dedication, even in the presence of fear and anxiety.

In an interview, Irina Aleksandrovna Viner, a prominent Russian rhythmic gymnastics coach, once stated, "When you are on the pedestal, you are the champion; when you step down, that's it—you are nothing and a nobody."[3] This quote has influenced my perspective and kept me disciplined even after my athletic career. Whether in moments of triumph or when stepping away from the spotlight, I was always reminded to stay grounded.

ENTERING THE ENTERTAINMENT INDUSTRY

With the strength and awareness I acquired, it seemed destiny was carving a clear path for me. I have always wanted to do more, and I'm constantly looking for the next challenge. About a year before I entered high school, an online advertisement caught my attention. It was a call from an agency seeking teenage girls to participate in the inaugural Miss Teen pageant. I read the requirements and thought, "This is tailor-made for me!" Bursting with enthusiasm, I printed the advertisement and dashed upstairs to find my parents. Waving the paper, I excitedly told them about the opportunity. Granted, standing at just 5'5", I fell a bit short of the traditional height requirements, but I was sure that my confidence, tenacity, and athletic prowess would make up for it. And indeed, they did.

I quickly found myself immersed in the world of pageantry, trying to captivate audiences on stage and in person for several years. Pursuing pageants parallel to athletic competitions taught me the importance of presenting myself eloquently and gracefully, regardless of circumstances.

There is a lot that happens behind the scenes in pageantry. It is not all about the beautiful dresses and the swimsuit category. I learned the art of commanding attention through speeches and developed a magnetism that captivated hearts and minds. It was a transformative experience, and the enhanced confidence and fortitude I gained from competing in pageants also improved my performance in gymnastics and beyond.

My father stepped in by spending hours formulating sample questions, drafting answers, and helping me understand the nuances of professional communication. He helped me memorize the responses and repeatedly practice them so that my words and expressions appeared natural over time. And he would remind me to stay "calme, gentille, intelligente," which translates from French as "calm, nice, and intelligent," a phrase he would repeat to me throughout my life. Meanwhile, my mother was busy altering dresses, coaching me in mastering the pageant walk, and choreographing the dance routine for the talent segment. Her efforts were crucial in securing my victory in the talent portion of the competition. Through these endeavors, my parents and I bonded, working together to position me for success.

Pageantry was my first foray into the entertainment industry. My goals were expansive, and I was eager to explore every facet of that world. Being a pre-eminent rhythmic gymnast made me appealing to modeling and acting agencies, and my parents supported me wholeheartedly, seeing my readiness to commit fully. They accompanied me to photoshoots, showcasing events, and auditions and sought opportunities that could propel my career within the industry. During one of the showcase events, I encountered an individual from New York who recognized the potential within me. He pointed out that someone possessing a triple-threat skill set like mine could be very successful in the entertainment industry.

My aspirations to become an actor, singer, and model in New York now burned bright. Over several months, I shuttled between New York and my gymnastics training commitments at home. I even dedicated time during a family road trip to working with my manager, attending auditions, participating in photoshoots, and creating polished video reels in Times Square that highlighted my dancing, acting, modeling, and interpersonal skills.

New York City offered ample opportunities, and I was fortunate enough to dance alongside renowned choreographers and audition for movies. Being hailed as a triple threat and "the next Selena Gomez," I had all the ingredients for success; all I had to do was keep up the momentum.

REFRAMING FAILURE

But fate had a cruel twist in store for me. Suddenly and inexplicably, I was cut from the Olympic pre-selection process, as the committee had already selected the gymnasts that they wanted for the Olympic training. It was a devastating blow, and it left me bewildered and disheartened. The reasons given were vague; all I knew was I was denied the opportunity to join the collective, and my individual career did not seem strong enough to pursue further. It felt as though my very soul had been pulled from my body.

I had reached a dead end.

No stranger to mental and physical adversity by now, I once again persevered. Each morning, tears streaming down my face, I found the strength to rise and go to the gym. Knowing that someone else would take my place if I didn't do it fueled my determination. So, I soldiered on for another year, pushing my body through demanding training sessions. However, as the injuries accumulated, and mentally I felt myself slipping away, the fire within me was slowly extinguished. My once-unshakable focus faded, and my motivation dissolved into a haze of doubt. The harsh reality settled in—I was training and working for a dream that had been snatched away.

During one rigorous gym session, we were preparing for Nationals. The heat was intense, and I was drenched in sweat. I had been dedicating hours to practicing a specific element, but frustration set in as I struggled to master it. My emotions boiled over, and I had a tantrum, crying and throwing my apparatus aside. I had hit my limit, and I couldn't concentrate any longer. What frightened me more was that I didn't even want to. Collapsing onto the carpet, I wiped the sweat from my forehead and removed my toe shoes, revealing the torn ball of my foot and a Band-Aid clinging precariously. The pain was second nature to me, and even though I probably needed stitches, my instinct was to soldier on—to wrap it up and persist, as I always had.

During my athletic career, I endured various ankle fractures and breaks, yet I still pushed myself to attend training. While I couldn't perform certain elements or complete full routines, I continued to train and learn new skills in a cast. Injuries were, in a sense, part of the package; a perfectly healthy professional athlete is an illusion. The body undergoes every possible experience on the path to reaching excellence.

After my breakdown, a choreography coach approached me on the carpet, asking how I was doing. With despair, I admitted, "I don't want to do this anymore." I decided to head home, knowing I was in no condition to train at that moment. However, the question of whether to continue with the sport at all remained.

In the end, after thirteen years of dedication to gymnastics, the universe made the choice for me. A major injury that had been ignored and brewing for years stripped me of everything I had. In an instant, I lost my athletic legacy, the fruits of all my labor, the potential career in New York, and the comforting routine that had defined my existence.

I once again felt abandoned and left with nothing.

For years, I carried the weight of shame and failure, unable to talk to anyone about the shattered pieces of my once-glorious dream. I had to abandon all my performing aspirations, as my injury greatly hindered my ability to dance and perform acrobatics, which had been among my defining skills and advantages. I wondered whether this injury had redirected my life entirely. If I hadn't been injured, could I have pursued a career in the entertainment industry? Would I have become an actress? A singer, maybe? I was too short for a modeling career: that much was evident, but I will never get an answer to my other questions. It's the lone mystery in my life.

But in hindsight, I realize that this setback was not a testament to my inadequacy but rather a pivotal moment that would shape my life in ways I couldn't have anticipated. It was the transition from my adolescence to adulthood. The injury was also a wake-up call, forcing me to confront the depth of my emotional investment in gymnastics. It was a bittersweet realization that the road ahead was no longer defined solely by medals and accolades but by the richness of personal growth and the pursuit of genuine fulfillment. I came to understand that I had my own identity beyond the boundaries of a sport.

I now see that my dream of making it to the Olympics was not just about competing there but also about the growth and learnings that unfolded along the way. The "failure" to reach the Olympics was merely one thread among countless others, each weaving together to form the intricate fabric of my life.

Following several months of rehabilitation, a window of opportunity emerged—a chance to focus on academics. I realized that with the discipline I possessed, I could redirect my energies toward any new pursuit.

We need to not be bound to a specific path, despite what societal pressures or self-imposed limitations may tell us. At any given moment, "[we] are one decision away from a completely different life."[4]

EMBRACING THE UNKNOWN

As I look back on this chapter in my life, I can't help but smile and feel grateful for the journey, even if it felt hard when I was in the moment, experiencing what I had to experience. Through all my years of dancing, athleticism, and creative expression, I have become a true embodiment of the art forms introduced to me.

I owe a debt of gratitude to my parents, whose dedication and attention to detail paved the way for my growth. Their belief in my potential and relentless support propelled me in this competitive world. They gave me the skill to thrive and the strong discipline and resilience that continue to shape my path.

But this chapter is not just about my accolades; it's about the lessons and skills I gained along the way. Each milestone, each performance, and each competition taught me something valuable about myself and the world around me.

The lesson that stands above the rest is that obstacles are inevitable regardless of the path we choose, and how we respond to them ultimately defines us. Some may give up at the first sign of a challenge, allowing their dreams to wither in the face of adversity, while some will push forward with steady determination. Moments of struggle and triumph shape who we are. And they did shape me. I have learned to embrace the unknown. So, which type of person will you be?

REFLECTIONS
ON DETERMINATION

For those who are still searching for that determination, know that finding it can take time. It's normal to have moments of doubt or to face challenges that make you question your resolve. Remember that determination isn't a constant state; it's something you can develop and strengthen over time. Here are some tips to help you harness and nurture your determination.

- Set clear goals, as having well-defined goals gives you a purpose and direction, making it easier to stay committed and accountable.
- Break large goals, which can be overwhelming, into smaller manageable steps. There is nothing wrong with taking one step at a time.
- Visualize your success, as this can boost your motivation. Imagine the feeling of accomplishing your goals and using it to fuel your determination.
- Surround yourself with supportive friends, family, or mentors who encourage you and provide perspective

during challenging times. Acquiring a reliant support system is a game changer.
- Celebrate your achievements and milestones, no matter how small they are. Acknowledging progress reinforces your commitment and motivates you.
- Be consistent. This is essential. Even on tough days, when you don't want to do anything, keep taking small steps toward your goals.

Life is full of unexpected twists and turns. But it's through these experiences that we discover who we are and what we are capable of. Embrace the challenges that come your way, for they hold the seeds of your growth within them. Allow yourself to be captivated by the dance of life, stepping boldly into the unknown, fully aware that with every stumble, you have the power to rise stronger and wiser.

In the symphony of existence, each of us possesses a unique melody to contribute. Nurture your passions, cultivate your talents, and never stop believing in your potential.

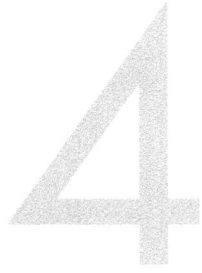

EPIPHANY: EMBRACING THE SHADOWS

["Epiphany": noun / i-ˈpi-fə-nē/]
An illuminating discovery, realization, or disclosure.[1]

THIS IS WHERE WE ENTER the convoluted depths of my young adulthood. In this chapter, I talk about a crossroad that I faced, and I show you how the relationships in my life led me there and what I learned from that pivotal moment.

Ah, relationships—the labyrinth of twisted emotions and expectations.

Growing up, I was convinced that love should be hard and earned. Tough love was the norm in my household, and I thought that was how things were meant to be. Little did I know the true magnitude of that belief back then. It served as a doorway to a multifaceted future, and stepping through it demanded that I confront the deep-seated generational strains that had silently governed my existence for years.

So, let's step through the doorway.

In trying to please my parents and make them proud, I followed their guidance blindly for about twenty years. I trusted them, as many kids do, believing they had answers to everything and that obeying them would bring me happiness. I think this pattern is all too common, and I was unaware there could be another way to live.

Individuals from non-Western backgrounds may feel torn between the values instilled by their cultures and the desire to embrace the Western ideals of self-fulfillment. They may be divided between loyalty to their cultural traditions and the desire to pursue personal happiness and self-actualization.

The clash of cultural values surrounding marriage and relationships exemplifies this difficulty. Many cultures view marriage as a cornerstone of life, a highly valued and deeply ingrained societal norm. They see it as a sacred bond that symbolizes commitment, stability, and family values. From a young age, individuals are taught that marriage is a significant milestone they should pursue earnestly.

In the culture in which I was raised, keeping a marriage alive is more important than individual desires or personal fulfillment. There is an emphasis on dedication, sacrifice, and endurance, even in the face of severe adversity. The concept of "until death do us part" holds immense weight; divorce is often stigmatized or seen as a last resort.

In contrast, the current Western mindset prioritizes personal happiness, individual autonomy, and self-fulfillment. The emphasis is on personal growth, pursuing one's passions, and finding a partner who aligns with one's own goals and aspirations. Leaving a relationship that no longer serves one's happiness is considered a valid choice and practice.

Let me be clear: I am grateful for the direction and care that my parents provided me with throughout my early years. Yet, in my youthful naivety, I was unaware of the repercussions of unquestioning loyalty to their beliefs or the views that were presented to me. It was only much later that I began to feel stuck in my self-made prison. I was a dormant volcano, with my true self flaming beneath the surface. The weight of my family's aspirations for me, influenced by our cultural customs and expectations, added more pressure.

I later realized how misguided, yet not unusual, it can be to prioritize parental approval so highly. The belief that love should be hard and that sacrifice and conformity were the ultimate keys to happiness became my misguided compass and subtly slowed down the blossoming of my own identity.

My aim in sharing my story is to serve as a guiding light for others who felt or feel similarly boxed in by helping them recognize that certain relationships, patterns, or individuals might not align with their well-being—and ultimately preventing them from making or continuing the same missteps I did. I am not seeking sympathy or harboring any vindictive motives; my sole purpose in sharing these events is educational.

A RELATIONSHIP FULL OF FOMO

As we know, life can shake us wide awake, sometimes in the rawest manner imaginable, prompting us to move on to the next phase in our lives. It's only at that moment that we fully comprehend the extent of the discomfort that comes with healing and understanding.

As I delved deeper in my early twenties into my psyche, I discovered various unexplored nuances; it felt as if a storm were raging within me. There came a point in my life when it seemed the weight of my challenges would never lift.

It all began when I found myself in a picturesque relationship with a man. Let's call him Sam.[2]

Our relationship was a source of sheer delight during the first few months. We connected effortlessly, enjoyed each other's presence, and reveled in shared moments. Sam displayed remarkable attentiveness, showered me with expensive gifts, and took me on memorable trips. However, as time progressed, I slowly removed the rose-colored glasses and learned of things that cast shadows over our connection. Regrettably, these revelations began leaving marks on our relationship.

After those first happy months, I began finding myself, night after night, going to bed consumed by sadness and waking up feeling dread. Yet, everyone around me made me believe that I had everything. I mean, it seemed as though I had it all on paper and on the canvas of social media. But behind closed doors, my reality had quickly become nightmarish.

Nobody knew the extent of my despair besides my counselor and Sarah and a few other close friends. I mostly hid it because "love is supposed to be hard," right? I didn't know any other way at that time; I was only twenty-two. My parents, particularly my mother, would emphasize that there was no cause for me not to feel happy. They'd point out that I possessed everything a girl could desire, suggesting that I might have been overly indulged and now could not value it fully. So, I often retreated into silence, suppressing my melancholy for months and years. I didn't want to appear ungrateful. I didn't want to be a disappointment in their eyes.

I can vividly recall the nights I would lie crumpled on the

cold bathroom floor. Curled in the fetal position, I would tightly embrace myself, rocking back and forth, whispering reassurances into the void. "You're going to be okay," I would repeat, hoping the words would somehow manifest as truth. Eventually, exhausted from the emotional turmoil, I would drift off to sleep, only to rise the next morning with a smile plastered across my face, ready to face the world once again. This pattern persisted for years until I reached a breaking point.

Experiencing intense emotions can force us to reflect on our values and why they seem to fail us—those poignant moments were the start of a path from which I could not turn back. I was growing tired of shedding tears on that bathroom floor while Sam was in the next room literally putting a barrier between us by closing the door and shaming me for my "self-imposed" isolation. He led me to believe that my nature and behavior caused him to isolate me and that I was solely to blame for these difficulties in our dynamic. Strangely, there was a kernel of truth there—I had, in fact, permitted this to persist because I didn't know how to assert myself or defend my worth in those moments.

I was utterly lost, with every avenue in my personal and professional life feeling like a dead end. Dissatisfaction consumed me, and it seemed as though no one truly comprehended the depths of my distress. I felt profound loneliness and retreated further into solitude.

I want to emphasize that individuals enduring any emotional mistreatment are not to blame for what they endure. The responsibility lies squarely on the shoulders of the individuals inflicting it. They are accountable for the words, behaviors, and actions that cause turmoil in another person. Perpetrators might employ emotional mistreatment tactics to assert control, satisfy their insecurities, or maintain a power dynamic within the relationship.[3]

In my opinion, Sam had many admirable qualities. He was hardworking, charming, dependable, adventurous, and resourceful. However, we later realized that we were opposites in every way. We had almost nothing in common. From my perspective now, we both feared being alone, so we relied heavily on each other for happiness instead of finding it within ourselves. I also acknowledge the role I played and that I was far from perfect in the relationship. There were times when I said or did things that inadvertently triggered him, contributing to the cycle of hurt between us. And despite my best efforts, I sometimes acted out, falling into the pattern of "hurt people, hurt people."[4]

This is a common dilemma for many couples, especially when they've invested significant time, money, and years of their lives into the relationship. It becomes difficult to walk away from such an investment, particularly if you're plagued by thoughts of "what if"—the sunk-cost fallacy.

That is where part of the concept of FOMO (fear of missing out) comes into play. It has become an ever-present specter in our modern lives. It lurks in the background, whispering anxiously in our ears. This fear permeates our day-to-day existence and seeps into the fabric of our personal and professional relationships. This fear compels us to say yes when we mean no, to overextend ourselves and sacrifice our well-being for the illusion of being part of every experience. It drives us to seek external validation, leading to continuous discontentment.

In long-term relationships, FOMO reflects the fear of unexplored paths. It lingers like a ghostly presence, making us question our choices. When we've been with someone for a long time and are unhappy, we wonder about the possibilities beyond our current relationship. But these thoughts can be full of guilt, particularly if we've invested a lot in that relationship. There are shared experiences, a life built together, and a comfortable and familiar bond. The fear of leaving all that behind can be paralyzing. So, we hesitate, afraid to make a decision that could alter the course of our lives, unsure if it's worth risking the stability we've cultivated.

We find ourselves caught between the fear of missing out on what could have been and the fear of losing what we already have. It becomes a delicate balancing act, juggling the longing for exploration with the desire for security.

But here's the truth: FOMO is a deceptive companion. Ultimately, you should determine the state and health of your relationship and if it satisfies you. The grass may be greener on the other side, but that doesn't mean you should jump ship at the first sign of difficulty, either. Relationships—like life itself—are a series of choices and trade-offs. By investing in your current partnership and establishing clear communication, you might open yourself up to the possibility of a deeper connection, growth, and beauty. However, not every relationship is worth saving. Only you know how you truly feel and what you want in your relationships. You have the power to advocate for yourself.

SETTLING

I always wanted to get married, or so I thought. I was, in a way, conditioned to think that I had to, so I made it into a target to accomplish by the time I was in my mid-twenties. I even gave Sam an ultimatum stating my target goals and my desired timelines. As a result, despite our disagreements, we got engaged after a few years, stubbornly moving forward with the "expected" steps.

The responsibility of wedding planning landed solely on me, and unconsciously, a deep resentment started to take root. I wasn't fully aware of what it was back then, but I sensed something was amiss. Nevertheless, I continued down that path because of my extreme sense of commitment. Our parents and friends approved and admired us on social media, where we presented a flawless image of our relationship. We had all the trappings of a comfortable life: a house, dogs, and regular vacations. Yet, beneath the surface, I was already deeply unhappy. And so was Sam. Despite our shared discontent, we were settling for each other out of fear and the familiarity of our routine.

So, what do I mean by "settling"?

Settling in a relationship is when individuals choose to remain in it despite their unhappiness or unfulfilled desires. It often occurs when fear, comfort, or external expectations outweigh the individual's happiness.[5] People may settle for various reasons, such as the fear of being alone, societal pressure to be in a committed relationship, financial dependency, or believing they won't find anyone better. In some cases, individuals convince themselves that their current situation is "good enough," even though deep down, they yearn for more.

And that was my narrative. Our narrative.

REFLECTIONS
ON RELATIONSHIP SATISFACTION

Performing regular check-ins on your current relationship or taking time to reflect on past ones is a valuable practice. To initiate your reflection, consider these key questions:

- Are you genuinely fulfilled and happy in this relationship?
- Are you proud to be in this relationship?
- Are your needs and desires being met?
- Are you heard and seen in the relationship?
- Do you feel a deep connection and compatibility with your partner?
- Are you settling because of fear or external pressures?
- How would you feel outside the relationship? Would anything significantly change?

It's crucial to be honest with yourself during this self-reflection process. Only you know how you truly feel.

If you've come to the realization that you might be settling or not where you expected to be in your relationship, you may want to explore addressing this when you're prepared, using the following suggested steps:

- Communicate openly and honestly with your partner about your feelings and concerns.
- Share your needs and desires and listen to their perspective as well. It's a two-way street.
- Together, explore whether there are any changes or compromises that could improve the relationship.
- Seek couples counseling and individual therapy for further insight and guidance (if necessary). Avoid bringing external opinions (friends, family, etc.) into the relationship.

Prioritize your happiness and well-being, and be prepared to make difficult decisions if necessary, such as pursuing individual growth or ending the relationship. Remember that everyone deserves to be in a relationship that brings them joy, fulfillment, and genuine happiness, whatever that looks like for you.

You may wonder why I chose to remain in a relationship despite my unhappiness. The truth is that fear was the driving force behind my decision. Remember when I mentioned how childhood shapes how we perceive the world, ourselves, and our relationships? For me, the seeds of doubting my self-worth had already been planted with the jokes my parents made about having to pay someone to love or marry me because of my hyper nature and strong opinions. Though these jokes were "innocent," and I truly believe they were intended to be completely harmless, they were still embedded into my psyche. I genuinely thought at that time that no man would ever love me for who I was and that settling for Sam was my only option.

A few weeks before the wedding, I vividly remember having a conversation with Sam that hinted at the true state of our relationship, and the last-minute wedding details that needed attention just added additional pressure. I was sitting on the couch while he was at the opposite end of the living room, as if we were trying to keep as much space between us as possible. There was an undeniable absence of warmth in the room.

I attempted to express my desire for us to write personal vows, some in my native language, to be recited after the conventional ceremony led by the officiant. This was the fourth time I had raised the subject. Sam responded with subtle disinterest as usual, and his gaze avoided mine.

The conversation continued the next day, but this time over text:

"You wanted us to write our own vows. You know I've been trying, eh?"

He continued, "I can't think of anything nice to say. What am I supposed to do? You demand that I say part of it in Russian. I literally have no motivation to do this."

I stared at my phone, disbelief washing over me, as I began crying.

"Where am I supposed to draw my inspiration from? Tell me."[6]

The texts became more painful: "Why am I even marrying you?" and "You don't deserve any vows." In his eyes, during miscommunications, I was a "bad girlfriend," and then I graduated to the "worst fiancée."[7] And you know what, I believe he really thought that. After all, we each hold our own standards, beliefs, and expectations. And, now, it is evident that I didn't meet his.

Yet, it makes me wonder, if he truly found me that inadequate as his future spouse, why did he stay with me? I have asked myself the same question since I felt similarly demoralized by him. The fact that both of us persisted only highlights the complex nature of relationships.

I felt bad for us.

Deep down, I knew something was wrong, but I kept suppressing my uncertainties.

Further sowing the seeds of self-doubt within me, everyone around me assured me that I just had cold feet, that this was normal—the pre-wedding blues. I simply clung to the hope that Sam would love me more once we were married and finally see me as enough.

Unfortunately, that hope was a naive one.

Typically, in social media and movies, we witness the excitement of brides-to-be celebrating with their bridesmaids in luxurious hotel rooms, wearing matching robes and sipping champagne. I had the opposite experience. The night before the wedding, Sarah and I shared moments of uneasy silence, and I found myself contemplating whether I should proceed with the marriage. We were both in our early twenties, lacking the wisdom to detect the "right" or "wrong" pre-wedding emotions. Sarah also brushed it off as cold feet, unaware of the depth of my inner chaos.

She sat on the couch in my bridal suite while I occupied the floor, and our eyes met. I mumbled, "Should I go through with this? Should I get married tomorrow? I'm not certain." I was thinking about the recent conversations between Sam and me, but I was already at the finish line. The wedding was just a day away, and I felt compelled to honor the commitment. The last thing I wanted was to cause embarrassment to our parents and their circle of acquaintances. After all, I appeared to have it all. What was wrong with me?

Before I continue, you may be familiar with the concept of red and green flags in a relationship. Green flags are indicators of a healthy and thriving relationship. These include open and effective communication, mutual respect and support, shared values and goals, trustworthiness, empathy, and emotional intelligence. A partner who actively listens to your concerns, encourages personal growth, and consistently shows kindness and understanding can display green flags.

On the other hand, red flags serve as warning signs of issues or behaviors that may damage a relationship. These can include dishonesty, manipulation, lack of respect, isolation, blame-shifting, possessiveness, lack of respect for boundaries, unwillingness to take responsibility for actions, and a pattern of controlling behavior. A partner who consistently dismisses your feelings, isolates you, or is unpredictable exhibits red flags.

Despite the red flags Sam and I both displayed in our relationship, the wedding continued as planned.

The morning of the wedding was filled with excitement as people applied their makeup and styled their hair, and the photographer captured precious moments. Babyshka diligently ironed her outfit, my sister took photos with her Polaroid camera, and my dress was proudly showcased for all to admire. Only one crucial element was missing—my happiness.

Guests were beginning to arrive, their smiles and excitement adding to the festive atmosphere. However, amid the cheerful commotion, my husband-to-be was delayed in arriving. Being somewhat superstitious, I couldn't help but view this as a sign, a final opportunity to reconsider my decision. Yet, I chose to proceed even with that perceived forewarning. I couldn't bear living with the "what if" and forever wondering about the path not taken.

Deep down, I knew that this was the beginning of the end. For months, I had told my family and friends that this didn't feel right. One time, I hid in my childhood bed, under the blankets in my parents' house, anxious about everything that was going on around me, but no one extended a hand. They thought I was unreasonable because they believed I had everything I could want.

So, there I was, getting ready to walk down the aisle, my

father beside me, proud and prepared to give me away. But I felt as though I had already disappointed him; I kept apologizing to him in my head, thinking, "I am going to leave this man, Apa. I am so sorry to make you do this. I am so sorry."

After the ceremony, according to our family's traditions, the bride and groom break bread, with the person who breaks the larger piece symbolically recognized as the "head" of the family. I happened to break the larger piece and felt a sense of triumph —my friend later commented, "When you broke that piece of bread, it felt as if you were unconsciously reclaiming control over your life." Hearing how others perceived my life was intriguing.

Anyway, it was a beautiful celebration; everything went as planned. Everyone was happy and had a good time. But I couldn't shake the anxiety that consumed me. I went through with it, yes, but instead of steady excitement, I felt unease as I awaited what the next chapter held for me.

As I had dreaded, during our honeymoon—a mere four days after our wedding—my husband uttered the words that sealed the fate of our marriage: "You're a bad wife."[8] It became clear that our wedding had not resolved anything; instead, it exacerbated the existing issues, legally binding us together in this deteriorating union.

I think it's not uncommon for individuals to find comfort in believing that marriage or starting a family will somehow heal the fractures and breathe new life into a faltering relationship. There's a widespread notion that these milestones can mend what's broken, offering a fresh start and renewed happiness. However, harsh reality often reveals that this is not the case.

Though it is traditionally viewed as a symbol of commitment and unity, marriage is not a cure-all for the fundamental issues within a relationship. While the ceremony itself can be a joyous celebration, it cannot resolve deep-rooted conflicts or ingrained patterns of dysfunction. In fact, the legally binding commitment of marriage can intensify pre-existing problems, adding pressure and complexity to an already fragile union. The hard truth is that a ceremony and a piece of paper cannot fix what is already broken.

In a similar vein, it's not wise to attempt to mend a failing relationship by enlarging one's family. The arrival of a child, in all its wonder and joy, ideally requires a solid foundation of love, trust, and mutual support. It can amplify existing tensions, as the demands of parenting often place additional pressure on an already strained connection, leaving both partners overwhelmed and further estranged.

The key to addressing a struggling relationship lies in confronting the issues head-on, outside of external factors such as marriage or children. It requires open and honest communication, a genuine commitment to personal growth, and a willingness to confront one's own flaws and shortcomings.

As Sam's upsetting label echoed in my mind, he asserted that, as his wife, it was my responsibility to ensure his happiness. But how could I make someone else happy, especially when my heart grew heavy with resentment? How could I fulfill this unreasonable task of bringing joy to someone's life when I felt depleted and emotionally wounded? It was clear that happiness could not flourish under such circumstances. The very idea of "making" someone happy felt suffocating.

This responsibility felt impossible. It seemed to dismiss the complex dynamics at play, neglecting the importance of mutual respect, understanding, and individual responsibility. Happiness, I believed, should not rest solely on the shoulders of one person. It should emerge from a collective effort, a shared commitment to nurturing each other's well-being.

EXIT STRATEGY

During the honeymoon, one evening in a restaurant, Sam and I continued our disagreements. At that moment, a wave of desperation washed over me, and I felt an overwhelming urge for someone, *anyone*, to witness the truth and understand the reality I was living.

That evening ignited something within me—a newfound determination to assert my voice, stand up for myself, and make choices that would shape my future. I realized that remaining silent and passive was no longer an option I was okay with.

This feeling continued for months until I couldn't tolerate it any longer. I even started to have nightmares. I dreamed of holding a small boy in my arms, with suitcases packed, standing before my husband, telling him to stay away. It was as if my subconscious was granting me a glimpse of what awaited me if I remained with my husband.

There are moments in life when we reach our breaking point, when we can no longer endure the weight of our circumstances. In these moments, we find the strength to change our destinies.

And so, I began working on a way out.

My first bold move was to resign from my managerial job to pursue my professional dreams. I was confident I could bounce back; however, it was not easy. Sam teased me during this transition, suggesting I apply for a job at a fast-food place when I had been out of work for only a week with no prominent leads.[9]

Despite his teasing, I kept going. I began to network with individuals who believed in me, even when I struggled to believe in myself. Their support became the foundation on which I rebuilt my shattered confidence. A few weeks later, I landed a new job and met people who would help me navigate my next steps to freedom.

I began to realize the power of my own abilities. I started to ask myself, If I can summon the strength to resign from my job and pursue my dreams, what's stopping me from leaving my marriage?

The snowball of empowerment started rolling. I realized that the mutable love I experienced in my childhood mirrored the "love" I received in my marriage. I had internalized the belief that love was supposed to be tough and that I should be grateful for any semblance of support or financial stability. But I learned the hard way that this was not love.

EMBRACING MASCULINE AND FEMININE ENERGIES

Even though I participated in pageants and was a rhythmic gymnast throughout my life, I endured criticism for not fitting into society's expectations of femininity. My mother played a significant part in instilling that viewpoint within me. I was labeled "too manly" and, at times, lacked the softness and delicacy necessary for successful relationships, and my assertiveness and ambition intimidated my partners. My identity seemed distorted and was used against me. The message was clear: a woman should not embody such qualities. When I tried asserting myself, my mother countered with remarks such as "No man would want to be with someone with such a dominant personality." Even when my competitiveness emerged, she advised me to use a softer approach, cautioning against competing with men on an equal footing. My mother emphasized the need to embrace more traditional femininity to avoid ending up alone, even linking my weight gain to a "masculine" build. And when she disapproved of something I did, she often commented, "Ouff, just like a man, Suzan."

While I now understand that she made these comments with the intention of "watching out for my best interests," as my father put it, I eventually told her how I felt about them. I forgave her for the sake of my personal growth, but I firmly rejected any similar comments moving forward.

What my closest circle failed to understand was that my assertiveness and energetic nature resulted from the challenges I had faced and the circumstances I had overcome. In a world that often felt overwhelming, I learned to rely on myself, to be self-sufficient and fiercely independent. My masculine energy became a survival mechanism, enabling me to create the stability and security I craved in my life that no one else could provide.

I became a pillar of strength, a force to be reckoned with. My self-reliance was born out of necessity, not out of a desire to defy societal norms or my parents. And yet, this strength was misconstrued, criticized, and misunderstood.

Deep down, I knew that my independence was not a flaw or a source of failure. As I looked inward, I discovered the transformative power of embracing both the divine feminine and masculine energies within me. Society often paints a picture of what it means to be a woman or a man, assigning rigid roles and expectations. But life can be about harnessing the divine feminine's nurturing and compassionate qualities while embracing the divine masculine's strength and assertiveness. By balancing these energies, I found wholeness and authenticity.

So, let's talk more about that.

Traditionally, society has assigned specific roles to men and women, dictating how they should behave and express themselves. Men have been expected to embody qualities associated with masculine energy, such as assertiveness, strength, and independence. On the other hand, women have been encouraged to embrace feminine energy, characterized by nurturing, empathy, and emotional sensitivity. Though limiting and confining, these roles have shaped the foundation of many relationships.

However, as we progress in society, these gender roles are being challenged. The modern-day understanding of feminine and masculine energy transcends biology and embraces the fluidity and diversity of human expression. We navigate a complex landscape where the balance between these roles and their encompassing energies can greatly impact our connections with others. Throughout history, individuals have consistently defied confined and inflexible gender norms. Fortunately, there is increasing recognition and embracing of authentic identities and how with people navigate their lives and relationships. It is an acknowledgment that each individual carries within themselves a unique blend of these energies, regardless of their gender identity.[10]

Both feminine and masculine energies have their strengths and contribute to the dynamics of a healthy partnership. In a modern relationship, the masculine and feminine energies dance together. In this relationship, both individuals can embrace their strengths and vulnerabilities, creating a safe space for growth and exploration.

This balance is not about conforming to stereotypes or following predefined roles. Instead, it is a celebration of the versatility of the human experience. It is about recognizing that both partners can embody qualities of both energies and find harmony in their unique blend.[11] The concepts of masculine and feminine energy are not inherently tied to a specific gender; individuals of any gender can access and embody both energies. And their expression can vary depending on circumstances and personal preferences.

REFLECTIONS
ON TAPPING INTO FEMININE AND MASCULINE ENERGIES

When you are in your feminine energy, you may notice that you:

- Have a heightened intuition and rely on your inner feelings to make decisions and navigate life.
- Are attuned to your emotions and allow yourself to experience and express them fully, without judgment or suppression.
- Are more flexible and adaptable in various situations. You may go with the flow and trust in the natural unfolding of events rather than try to force or control outcomes.
- Are receptive to others' support, love, and nurturing.
- Embrace and celebrate your sensuality by finding joy and pleasure in sensory experiences.

- Prioritize building and nurturing different types of relationships and connections.
- Tap into your creative impulses, and you may find joy in art, music, writing, or any other form of creative exploration.
- Embrace being in the present and find beauty in the simplicity of life.

When you are in your masculine energy, you may:

- Have a strong drive and determination to set and achieve goals. You may be results-driven and strive for success in various areas of your life.
- Prioritize rationality, logic, and critical thinking. You may excel at problem-solving and making decisions based on facts and evidence. You may have a solution-oriented mindset, tackling challenges head-on.
- Have strong self-assurance and be comfortable asserting your ideas, opinions, and boundaries.
- Value your autonomy and enjoy taking responsibility for your actions and outcomes as you prefer to rely on your skills and resources.
- Take charge, assume leadership roles, initiate action, organize tasks, and inspire others to achieve shared objectives.
- Prefer a linear, step-by-step approach to tasks and projects. You may thrive in structured environments and be skilled at planning, organizing, and executing ideas.
- Rely on reason and logic, weighing pros and cons objectively. Emotions may play a lesser role as you prioritize practicality and efficiency.

I noticed that my line of work demanded considerable masculine energy from me. I needed to be assertive, a problem-solver, and proactive to thrive in that setting. However, this experience also led me to understand the importance of balancing the masculine and feminine energies in my life. When I returned home, I yearned to embrace my feminine energy to restore equilibrium within myself. Yet, within the context of my marriage, maintaining a balance between masculine and feminine energies became nearly impossible; hence, I leaned toward my masculine energy to survive.

I learned the hard way that staying exclusively in one's masculine energy for extended periods can harm our overall well-being. While masculine energy has its strengths and benefits, maintaining an imbalance by neglecting the feminine aspects within us can lead to physical, mental, and emotional health issues. As recent studies indicate, adhering to a single energy archetype is not ideal, and concepts such as toxic femininity and toxic masculinity now bring more awareness to these important dynamics.[12]

At the beginning of our relationship, our "roles" were clearly defined. Sam supported us financially while I focused on maintaining the house and being a full-time student. However, when I started working full-time while still pursuing my studies, there was an unspoken assumption that the household duties mostly remained my responsibility.

For months, I tried to establish a fair division of tasks in our relationship. Despite my best intentions, whatever I did was never quite right. I constantly second-guessed my actions, trying desperately to meet his expectations yet always coming up short. It was disheartening; no matter how hard I tried, I could never earn his approval or the recognition I craved.

At the same time, my new financial independence diminished Sam's monetary influence on our relationship. I realized I could now choose and create my desired circumstances, and I began asserting myself and voicing my independence. That, on its own, added fuel to the fire.

PUTTING DOWN THE CHECKLIST

Life has a way of orchestrating unexpected events that catalyze our personal awakening. Through these trials, we embark on a self-discovery journey and recognize our self-worth. It is a deeply individualistic process that unfolds over time, revealing its treasures gradually, like a blossoming flower.

I hope that the few lessons I shared serve as guiding beacons for those who find themselves in similar situations. The most important of these lessons is that self-worth and self-doubt are intertwined, and we must recognize that our worth is inherent and independent of external validation. The checklist mentality, driven by fear of the unknown, can only lead to a contentless life. As I mentioned in the introduction, that was precisely the path I followed in my early life. By age twenty-five, I had diligently ticked off all the items on my comprehensive checklist of life achievements, yet I felt hollow and unfulfilled.

Living with a checklist mentality means structuring your life around predefined goals, societal expectations, and a "nonnegotiable" path to success. This approach often involves pursuing accomplishments that are considered conventional markers of achievement: getting a certain degree, landing a prestigious job, finding a partner, buying a home, making a certain amount of money, and so on. While these goals are not inherently negative, problems arise if you pursue them solely to check them off, without considering personal values, passions, or genuine aspirations, or only to make someone else happy.

Individuals living with a checklist mentality might find themselves on a constant quest to fulfill predetermined criteria. Their lives can feel automated, detached from their authentic desires, and lacking in fulfillment. As achievements are unlocked and checkboxes marked, the initial euphoria quickly fades, leaving an emptiness stemming from the realization that external signs of success don't necessarily equate to true happiness or a sense of purpose.

Living with a checklist mentality can also lead to many successes as you learn to be hyper-organized and productive with your time despite causing a disconnection from your authentic self. After twenty-seven years, I was able to find a balance by embracing a more reflective approach that values self-awareness, personal growth, and alignment with my core values. This way, when I begin pursuing new goals, they are infused with purpose and a desire for a more meaningful and fulfilling life.

Self-love and self-worth are not destinations reached overnight. They are the products of an ongoing, ever-evolving process. So, if you find yourself at the beginning of your awakening, remember that this is just the starting point. Be prepared for the unexpected and for the challenges that lie ahead. Trust in the process, knowing that you are still moving forward even when you're taking steps backward.

This part of my story was a testament to the human spirit's resilience and ability to grow and transform. Naively, I thought the challenges I had already faced were the summit of my journey. Little did I know that these were only the first steps toward a more profound understanding of my inherent worth. Life had more tests in store for me before I could fully embrace my shadows.

This was only the beginning of my epiphany.

5

~~LAMENTATION:~~ THE UNVEILED CYCLE

["Lamentation": noun / ˌla-mən-ˈtā-shən/]
An expression of sorrow, mourning, or regret: an act or instance of lamenting.[1]

LIFE HAS A FUNNY WAY of showing us its true colors; it sneaks up on us when we think we've overcome our darkest moments, revealing new challenges. That's the thing about awakenings—they're not one-time events that miraculously solve all our problems. No, it is a challenging process.

My struggles with my new reality didn't magically vanish, but here's the upside: I had begun to change. My perspective had started to shift, and I no longer succumbed to adversity without question or action. The turning point came when I realized I deserved more than the life I had been conditioned to accept or build. The circumstances I had allowed to unfold did not reflect my worth. They were mere stepping stones toward understanding myself and my purpose.

One thing life has taught me is that the cycle of difficulties will continue no matter what we do. By accepting this fact, I have begun to find peace. The lessons I had gathered from past experiences became my beacon of light, illuminating the path before me. What once seemed impossible now appeared conquerable.

I love this quote often attributed to Bob Marley: "You never know how strong you are, until being strong is your only choice."[2] I believed in those words, and I entered unfamiliar territory with that belief.

BREAKING POINT

Around half a year after the wedding, the shaky environment at home was starting to impact every aspect of my life. No matter where I went, whether for work or leisure, I had emotional breakdowns. To try to cope, I changed my appearance by cutting my hair short. It was a desperate attempt to find some temporary relief, but it only made me feel worse about myself.

I felt mentally, emotionally, and physically defeated. During a work event, my colleagues noticed that something was off. They remembered me from a year ago, full of energy and ready to take on the world. But now, I seemed to be merely surviving each minute.

Their observations were accurate, and it saddened me that I couldn't hide my feelings anymore. When a colleague pulled me aside and asked how I was doing, I broke down, crying and venting about everything I was emotionally going through. I explained how I knew that I would be solo by next year and starting my life anew. It felt as if my heart were about to burst from my chest, and I realized that this meltdown was a cry for change, a final push to prioritize myself.

I did not want to remain trapped in an unhappy marriage. I did not want to see myself become a shattered version of who I truly was, clinging to fragments of hope and living a façade.

After returning from the event, I went to dinner with Sarah. "What's wrong?" she asked, the moment she settled into the car.

I replied curtly, "Not now," and we silently proceeded to the restaurant.

Inside the restaurant, Sarah still looked concerned. I began to open up about my decision to end my marriage and my commitment to follow through with it.

"I'm done, Sarah. I can't continue. It's just not possible," I said, sighing.

"Then don't," she replied. No second-guessing, no judgment, just all the love and support I needed.

We sat in silence until our orders were placed.

"What's your plan now?" she asked.

"I'll start by informing my parents and then seeking resources to break free." I leaned against the table, propping up my elbows and resting my head in my hands, overwhelmed by despair. "Ugh, our lives are so intertwined, but I must take that first step. I'll figure it out as I go."

"Figuring things out has always been your forte, Suz. It's your strength. You're Suzanna Alsayed, after all."

We laughed. She was right. It was indeed my strength, and

the time had come to channel it into extracting myself from this situation.

"Listen, no matter what you decide, my door is open. You're welcome to stay for as long as you need until you chart your next path," she assured me.

It was an immense relief to know I had a place to turn to when—not if—I took that step.

With that, I began working on the separation process, choosing to prioritize my well-being.

Summoning all my courage, I knew the next step would be to tell my parents about my decision. I hoped they would understand and back me. Unfortunately, their reaction was the opposite, leaving me feeling as if I had been abandoned once again—this time as an adult.

But I had firmly decided, and I no longer cared if I lost people around me for it. It was me against the world.

Amid this upheaval, someone unexpected entered my life—Chuck. He provided support and guidance through challenges I had never expected to face at such a young age, becoming an uncle figure to me.

Chuck and I formed an instant bond. We viewed life through a shared lens despite our large age difference. In Chuck, I found a refuge I hadn't encountered in a long time. I could pour out my thoughts without restraint, and he always offered an attentive ear. One day, during a road trip for work, we had a long heart-to-heart about my recent decision that solidified our friendship. As hours slipped by, I vented, and he listened. He also revealed his own experiences, telling me that he had gone through similar challenges in his youth.

"I feel like I've hit a dead end. It's like I'm trapped in a relentless cycle of misery," I confessed, gazing out the car window.

"Before you initiate the process, think through every aspect and possible outcome," he said. "Make sure you've explored all possibilities. But I know you, Suzanna. You're diligent and think fast, like a Ferrari. I bet you've already scrutinized it all." He laughed.

"Oh, I definitely have. I even put together a massive list weighing the pros and cons," I joked, a hint of a smile forming.

"Of course you did. Easy paths were never your style anyway."

Chuck was similar to Sarah; he always listened, shared his wisdom, offered candid opinions, and withheld judgment, and that was exactly what I needed. From that car ride onward, he became my supporter by being there through every major life decision for years to come.

This experience taught me a valuable lesson: family is not solely defined by blood. There are individuals who genuinely understand and care about you, sometimes even more than your kin.

THREE MORE MONTHS

To my dismay, influenced by their old-fashioned beliefs and their perception of who I was, my parents were against my dissolving the marriage. It often felt like they still saw me, particularly my mother, as the eighteen-year-old version of myself who lived under their roof.

During a holiday, while I was writing an article for a magazine, my family sat together on the couch watching TV. I had my laptop open on my lap, and my mother asked what I was working on. I said that I was working on submitting an article that was longer than the required word count.

"I am cutting some words down to meet the guidelines," I said, pressing the delete button.

She responded, "Remember when your early high school teacher commented on your tendency to ramble and write overly long essays? It seems like nothing has changed."[3]

I could feel myself flaring up, but I decided not to react. I couldn't understand why my mother had brought up such an old reference instead of celebrating or being interested in what I was trying to achieve. My high school experiences were not at all relevant.

Whether the topic was household responsibilities, cooking, relationships, or day-to-day life, my mother often focused on my shortcomings and areas of improvement instead of recognizing my progress and positive transformations. Each time, it was clear that she didn't know who I had become or wanted to be.

My parents believed it would be difficult for me to move on from my marriage, especially since I was accustomed to a life of comfort. I seemed to have it all in their eyes, so why would I want to escape that? They blamed me for my unhappiness and for not finding a way to make the marriage work.

Despite all my personal growth and newfound strength, the influence of my parents and my partner still weighed heavily on me. At that time, I still craved their approval. My parents even cooperated with my husband to convince me to keep trying in the marriage, assuring me that if I fulfilled three extra conditions, he would magically transform into the husband of my dreams. In their eyes, and even in his, I was the source of all the misery. Still, I fell for their assurances. Even then, the "what if" was still haunting me. What if I leave too early? What if I haven't done everything I can to salvage the marriage? What if I do what they say and Sam does become the husband of my dreams?

I did everything they asked, but nothing changed; I only wasted three more months.

The last attempt to keep the marriage alive was a vacation. And that ended up being the breaking point.

We didn't share a bed or a single civil conversation. Sam would occasionally joke that our photos at various landmarks would be used for our future online dating profiles. Occasionally, he would boast about his ability to attract other partners effortlessly once I wasn't in the picture anymore. One evening, when we were having dinner, he reiterated that we had nothing in common and was baffled that we still got married.[4]

I allowed him to revel in his trivial triumphs because, despite the opinions that everyone had regarding our marriage, I was determined to escape. I knew I had to tolerate it for a bit more time. My perspective had already evolved to thinking about "when" I would depart, not "if," and I was taking the necessary steps to leave with my dignity intact.

On our way home from the vacation, our plane encountered mechanical difficulties an hour into the flight, somewhere over the vast ocean. As the flight attendants informed us that we would need to make an emergency landing, I thought: "I do not wish to depart this world beside someone I don't love anymore." I was shocked at my bluntness and thoughts—and extremely relieved when we landed safely.

Two weeks later, I served Sam with divorce papers.

I left everything and shielded myself from everyone who did not support me for the sake of my sanity and happiness.

I've come to understand that, at that time, my parents and Sam perceived me not as a true reflection of who I was or am but rather as a reflection of themselves. Nobody can fully understand your emotions or all the details of your life. If you fail to take action, no one else will step in on your behalf or disrupt your existing patterns.

INDEPENDENCE

I handled the divorce alone. I immersed myself in the study of family law, assets, and the best practices for navigating the complexities of the legal system. I went to court, orchestrated the process from beginning to end, and resigned everything to Sam. The only thing I made sure to retain at any cost was the custody of our dogs, my happiness in the form of fur.

I abandoned my entire way of life; none of it was important to me anymore. It had all been superficial. What truly mattered was cultivating self-love and discovering my authentic self, untouched by the influence of others. I knew I would acquire all the material things again, but this time, it would be through my own efforts. The "it" inside me that I'd had since childhood—a resilient force that nurtured my confidence—kept reassuring me.

I knew I would be more than okay.

During the divorce proceedings, I discovered I had been ignorant of key details about our daily lives. I had little knowledge regarding our financial status, shared asset ownership, and even the details for bill payments and tax filings. Following our separation, I even thanked Sam for the financial efforts and responsibilities he shouldered.

My marriage and its ending taught me that in relationships built on mutual trust and respect, making practical arrangements that underpin a shared life can offer security for everyone involved. Love is undeniably beautiful, but life is full of unexpected twists. Foreseeing how someone close to you might evolve or respond to life's challenges is impossible. Now, let me be clear: the worst doesn't always happen, but it's prudent to exercise caution. Safeguarding your interests and well-being in any relationship is a wise choice.

Creating a foundation of trust, fostering open communication, and establishing boundaries can protect both partners. This approach allows love to flourish, all while knowing you've taken steps to ensure your security and happiness.

REFLECTIONS
ON CREATING A SHARED LIFE

When making major life decisions such as moving in together, purchasing assets, getting married, or having children, have open and honest discussions with your partner. Here are some key topics you can consider to prompt discussion:

Take the time to understand each other's core values and beliefs. Discuss what matters most to each of you regarding relationships, family, and personal and professional goals. Identify areas of alignment and potential areas of compromise.

Explore your cultural backgrounds and traditions. Discuss how you both want to incorporate these aspects into your shared life. Consider how cultural differences may impact your daily routines, celebrations, and interactions with family and friends. An example I frequently share with people in my life is the choice of which family's holiday celebrations to attend. What might the conversation look like, and what strategies can be used to reach a compromise?

Share your religious or spiritual beliefs and any political views you hold. Discuss how these principles may affect your decisions as a couple and how you envision incorporating or reconciling any differences. I habitually pose this hypothetical scenario to my friends: What if both of your countries were involved in a conflict or a religious uprising between your respective faiths occurred? How would you preserve harmony and mutual respect in your relationship?

Be transparent about your financial situation, including income, debts, and expenses. Discuss your stances toward money, budgeting styles, and long-term financial goals. Consider how you will handle joint finances, savings, loans, credit, investments, and any obligations you may have that occurred before and during the relationship.

Clearly define the roles and responsibilities each of you will have in the household. Consider how you will divide tasks such as cooking, cleaning, and other chores and responsibilities. Establishing expectations and finding a balance will help avoid conflicts in the future.

Talk about the importance of having a strong support system. Identify your support networks, including friends, family, and community. Discuss how you can lean on and involve these support systems as you navigate major life events together.

Discuss potential challenges and setbacks. This is crucial because life is unpredictable. Talk about your contingency plans for unexpected situations such as job loss, health issues, or financial difficulties. A backup plan can provide reassurance and help you feel more secure in your decisions.

Talk about an exit plan. This may not be the most romantic topic, but it's essential. Discuss what would happen if your relationship were to face irreparable difficulties. Talk about how you would handle separation or divorce, including asset division and potential custody arrangements if you have children.

Creating written agreements and plans can benefit you and your partner beyond the possibility of separation. It is also a precaution in case one partner faces illness, incapacity, or even death.

The specifics of these agreements may vary depending on your geographical location, environment, and available resources. The circumstances and frameworks that apply to you can influence the detail and complexity required to document these plans.

Maintaining one's independence can benefit both individuals in a relationship. This is particularly important for women, as they can become more vulnerable and inclined to stay in an unhappy environment, prioritizing their survival (and potentially the survival of dependents) and well-being.[5] Fostering educational or financial independence helps establish a more equitable dynamic between partners and maintains a balanced level of respect. The type and level of independence you want will also depend on your circumstances. In my experience, the preliminary financial independence I gained let me explore new opportunities and life paths outside my marriage. As a result, I promised myself I would never be in such a vulnerable position again.

I am happy that I honored the conditions and tried for those last few months of my marriage—it was my final test. Those ultimatums freed me from the uncertainties, "what ifs," and doubts that plagued me.

I believe Sam and I exhausted all possible efforts to salvage the marriage; despite all our attempts, the relationship remained unfixable. Most importantly, I no longer wanted to mend it either. Regardless of the consequences, I wanted to move on.

Run away, actually.

Solitude became an upgrade in my life, liberating me from the expectations of others, who met my decision with discontent, failing to see the depths of my emotions and the complexities of my life. I grew tired of having to convince people that this change was necessary. I knew my reasons, and that was sufficient for me.

There comes a point for each of us when we begin to outgrow partners, friends, and even family members, and this was my moment.

Sarah, Chuck, and Babyshka provided me with consistency during that phase of my life. Sarah opened her home to me; Chuck was always there to chat, while Babyshka became a solid pillar of support for my emotional well-being. Babyshka's daily calls were my primary source of familial support. Even when I lacked the energy to answer the phone and engage in conversation, she left me heartfelt voicemails. She understood that my simply knowing she was there for me brought immense comfort. To this day, I have kept all those voice notes as a cherished reminder of her care.

In one of my favorite voicemails, she said, "You know, Suzanna, I forgot that I once went through a similar situation when I was younger, just like you. But as time goes on, those memories fade away. You'll come across someone wonderful. All right, take care. Love you. Bye, Babyshka." It made me smile whenever she said it was her, as if I couldn't tell.

Divorce was more than just the end of a relationship for me; it was when I embraced the unknown with open arms. I shed the shackles of old expectations and defined my own path.

During that time, I believed leaving would be the hardest part of my adult life, but it turned out to be one of the easiest.

TEMPORARY COMPANIONSHIP

Even though I welcomed solitude, I lacked the knowledge to navigate it and did not know what was healthy and what was not. The concept of being alone as an adult was unfamiliar to me, and I had never sought it out nor desired it before.

Conveniently, I was introduced to Paul.[6]

Paul's presence in my life made me realize that we encounter many individuals who are only with us for a season, gracing our lives briefly. It is crucial for us to accept the temporary nature of these connections. Though it may not always be easy, we must find comfort in the fact that people come and go as part of the unpredictable rhythm of life. Each encounter, regardless of its duration, may hold significant lessons. Just as the seasons change, so do the people we meet.

Paul entered my life quickly and departed just as swiftly, yet he left a lasting impression. His focus on his career was inspiring, and he recognized untapped potential within me. He was exactly who and what I needed after my divorce.

"Suzanna, do you realize that you're a remarkably talented writer?" he would state while reading my work and publications. He was the one who helped me recognize just how much I love writing.

He was eager to pool resources, showing me how it is possible to gain financial success by harnessing one's strengths, and introduced me to entrepreneurship. Under Paul's influence, I was motivated to elevate myself further. We shared similar ambitions, dedication, and a mutual aspiration to build a "small empire" one day. Our dynamic radiated an entirely different energy from the one I felt with with my former husband—polar opposites.

I quickly became accustomed to the rapid pace of our relationship. In fact, my life had always seemed to operate at a different rhythm than that of those around me. But this time, it was due to outside influences.

A global pandemic hit—an event I never anticipated in our modern era. As a disaster and emergency management academic and practitioner, I was consumed by the implications in my every waking hour. Each day brought unprecedented challenges. Railway blockages, supply chain disruptions, toilet paper shortages, panic-driven hoarding, power outages, fear of getting the virus, devastating explosions, vaccines, and even natural disasters further compounded the chaos. It felt as if the apocalypse were near.

As government directives grew increasingly restrictive, Paul and I faced a pivotal decision: to isolate together or bring our relationship to an end.

Consequently, I found myself moving once again. And then, the world came to an abrupt halt as lockdown measures took effect.

But remember, I was still in the middle of a divorce, a process that required filing documents in court.

The divorce proceedings were complex. I had to wake up in the middle of the night, several times a week, to line up outside the courthouse by 4:00 a.m., hoping to secure a spot inside when the doors opened at 8:00 a.m. and then make it to work on time. Social distancing measures meant that the waiting area had limited capacity, resulting in a long line that wrapped around the building. People stood patiently, donning masks, maintaining a distance of two feet from one another, wrapped in blankets; some even brought foldable chairs for comfort, clutching lunch bags and thermoses of coffee. We knew we were in for an extended wait.

While I stood in that line, I overheard numerous tales of bitter divorces, intense child custody battles, fraud cases, and tragic accidents resulting in losing loved ones. I felt grateful for the relative simplicity of my circumstances—"just" a divorce. It was humbling to see the struggles faced by others while remembering that, despite the challenges of my personal life and the global pandemic, I still had the fortune of being employed and having a safety net, my health, and the opportunity for a fresh start.

Somehow, though, I knew this calmness was destined to be temporary. My intuition hinted that something was stirring in the background.

I wish my intuition had been wrong.

ENDURANCE TEST

Babyshka began exhibiting worrisome symptoms—a sudden fever spike and a persistent cough. We were initially concerned she had contracted the virus that was spreading all over the world. Strangely enough, we found ourselves wishing it were just that. The reality soon proved to be far worse.

Babyshka was rushed to the hospital, and we could only worry from home due to the strict pandemic restrictions. Only my mother was granted entry because Babyshka did not speak English, and even her presence was restricted; my mother was informed that she had to leave shortly after arriving. The subsequent communication with the medical staff would be solely through phone calls or video chats facilitated by an iPad.

Left alone in the hospital, Babyshka endured a two-day wait

until her diagnosis was confirmed. She received a Stage 4 pancreatic cancer diagnosis—a devastating blow.

Normally, she would visit the doctor yearly for routine check-ups. Unfortunately, due to the pandemic, she'd had to skip her annual visit that year, and it turned out to be the visit that could have made a significant difference in her health and chances.

The shocking news of Babyshka's terminal cancer diagnosis was delivered to us over the phone, and it became our responsibility to convey this heartbreaking information to Babyshka herself due to the language barrier. I vividly recall the three of us —my father, mother, and me—gathered in the basement with the phone in the center of our coffee table put on speaker. Somehow, I took on the role of spokesperson with the doctor. At the same time, my mother translated the message to Babyshka, and my father listened attentively to ensure the medical diagnosis that was communicated was understood by everyone. We took turns speaking in three different languages, doing our best to understand the gravity of the situation.

Initially, we were hesitant about delivering such news over the phone. It seemed so heartless, but circumstances left us no choice. The medical staff then decided to call us on the iPad so we could at least see Babyshka.

When we finally shared the news with Babyshka, her face grew pale almost immediately as she realized that her life was approaching an abrupt standstill. The only question that Babyshka asked was for my father.

"Is there no chance?" she whispered softly, almost to herself.

We just looked at each other and then observed Babyshka via the iPad screen, sitting in a state of shock.

"We will try our best," my father replied in a gentle tone.

We all felt helpless. That moment remains etched in my memory, as she was never quite the same after receiving the diagnosis.

The fact that we could not visit Babyshka in the hospital due to the pandemic protocols added to our distress. We longed to be by her side during such a challenging time. Witnessing the deterioration of this beautiful and positive woman who played a motherly role in my life was incredibly difficult, especially since there was little we could do to alleviate her suffering and reverse the course of her illness.

During that period, Chuck and his wife were a source of moral support, providing my family with the latest updates on the ever-changing protocols. Chuck had stood by my side during my divorce and was now helping me face Babyshka's life-altering diagnosis.

I had daily check-in video calls with Chuck, where he would ask about her well-being and my emotional state. During one of these calls, a few days after the last time I saw Babyshka in person, I said, "The fact that I can't just go and see her is tearing me apart. She's all alone in the hospital, and we can't even be there for her. I feel powerless, missing her so much and wishing I could do more. It's not fair for her to go through this. I don't even know how to process all of this anymore."

Chuck released a sympathetic sigh and said, "I understand this is incredibly difficult, especially given your inclination to organize and control things. So, it's especially challenging to cope with something that's completely beyond your influence."

As I nodded, my emotions took over, and tears began to flow.

"Suzanna, try to view this from a perspective of gratitude," he said. "I realize it's tough, but not everyone can say they've had someone like Babyshka in their lives. Not everyone has been fortunate enough to experience such a pure presence—someone who loves them unconditionally. You're genuinely lucky."

Though I was still crying, I was touched by his words.

He continued, "Despite the current state of the world, you're putting forth your best effort. Don't burden yourself with so much pressure. You'll be able to see her again. Babyshka is resilient, and she'll remain strong for you. Remember, having a loving granddaughter like you is also a blessing for her. You share great fortune in having each other."

It was true that by then, Babyshka and I had shared a lifetime of experiences together.

After a few weeks, Babyshka was finally released home, and nurses would visit daily to monitor her condition and administer medications. Despite the pandemic restrictions on travel, work commitments, and household limits, I spent as much time as possible with her at my parents' house.

On one visit, Babyshka expressed her deepest desire: "I wish I could see you become a mother and have children. I know I'm going to miss out on that. Oh, how I wish I didn't have to miss it." Those words pierced me to the core. They still do because it pains me to think that if I had ended my marriage earlier, I could have found someone to build a family with on a solid foundation, and Babyshka could have been a part of that experience.

It was heartbreaking to see her enduring so much pain. I couldn't help but feel that she deserved so much more than life had dealt her. If only I could have taken away her suffering and made everything better for her.

Meanwhile, my life remained disorderly. Paul and I faced our own challenges, and we found it difficult to support each other while simultaneously dealing with our struggles. We became like roommates, and the quarantine protocols may have been the sole factor holding us together. We fell into a pattern and followed a routine of working side by side for twelve to eighteen hours a day, eating individually at our desks, occasionally sharing some business insights, perhaps exchanging a few words while walking the dogs, and retiring to separate beds.

Paul stood by my side during that time, but as he had his own difficulties, his presence gradually transformed from a source of comfort to more of a burden. And I believe he might have felt the same about me. Both of us seemed to be trapped in survival mode, unable to spend extended periods alone to find temporary solace.

Life was coming at me from every corner. I was juggling a divorce, navigating the professional and personal impacts of a global pandemic, trying not to contract the virus, and facing entrepreneurial challenges, all while building a business from scratch. I was also constantly worried about Babyshka's deteriorating health and the limited time we had left with her, all while trying to determine and solidify the next steps in my life.

Each day seemed like a test of endurance, with overwhelming trials demanding my attention. The weight of them all was immense, and overcoming them was an uphill battle. It felt like a never-ending cycle without any relief or chance to catch my breath.

LOSING MY ANCHOR

As Babyshka's condition worsened, the decision was made to transfer her to palliative care. We were grateful that her room was on the first floor, with a window that became a source of connection for us. My mother, sister, and I, accompanied by my two dogs, would frequently gather outside the hospital window, attempting to communicate with her through the phone. This way, she could at least see us and hear our voices, even though her speaking ability had greatly diminished. Although we could see her reactions, all we wanted was to hug her. We were so close, yet so far.

At last, one day, my mother and I received permission to visit Babyshka the following day. I couldn't wait; I even planned to work from the hospital and keep her company.

That day, my mother called me around 8:05 a.m. to say she was about to enter the hospital. She gave me parking instructions and asked when I would be arriving. I was preparing my laptop and assured her I would be there around 8:30 a.m.

Less than five minutes later, my phone rang again; this time, my mother's voice was filled with distress. "I was too late," she cried. "I am too late. Babyshka died. I didn't make it in time. I was too late."

Everything in my life suddenly stopped. Once again, I

couldn't remember how to breathe. It felt as if I were back at the train station as a child.

The frailty of life had revealed itself. Just three months after her diagnosis, I lost the person who meant the world to me. A part of my soul died alongside her.

Adding to my grief, the complexities around me persisted; Paul unexpectedly concluded our relationship the day after Babyshka's passing. He simply didn't want to carry on and sought solitude. Much like many other things at that time, he swiftly exited my life. Then, shortly after that, four other extended family members succumbed to the grasp of the pandemic. We've all heard it before: "When it rains, it pours."[7]

I was left without words; the magnitude of it all was overwhelming.

Even though we had both moved on, Sam attended Babyshka's funeral. Seeing him there, shedding tears alongside my family and paying his respects to a woman who had been a kind presence in his life for half a decade, brought closure to me.

I was happy for him. For us. At that moment, my sole wish for him was to find happiness. We both deserved it.

And that was the last time I saw him.

After the funeral, I sat alone in a quiet park, numb. I felt scattered and confused, and once again, I found myself starting over. I desperately needed to make big changes in my life, but how? I was already holding on by a thread.

In the aftermath of Babyshka's death and another breakup, I learned a hard lesson about the consequences of my actions. I realized that instead of reflecting on my own, I had been jumping from one relationship to another. I was afraid to feel unwanted, so I didn't give myself time to heal and discover the root of my troubles.

I had made the same mistakes with Paul that I'd made with Sam. I hadn't learned from my past experiences.

It felt like déjà vu.

In fact, these patterns would continue until I acknowledged them, learned from them, and made the necessary changes.

That is the beauty of karma.

Just when I believed I had "unveiled the cycle" and moved beyond the lessons I needed to learn, I confronted the sobering truth that the cycle had not been completed and there were more lessons to be revealed.

I was in for another ride.

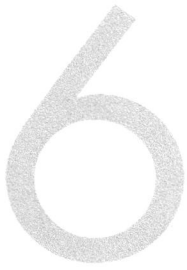

~~FORELSKET:~~ THE SPELLBINDING WALTZ

["Forelske seg": phrasal verb]
Fall for: to fall in love with (someone).[1]

I FOUND MYSELF NEWLY SINGLE, once again in a position to work on myself. This time, I consciously decided to keep an open mind and explore the world's possibilities.

I had experienced disappointment in multiple relationships, lost loved ones, moved several times, and dealt with the ongoing pandemic. On top of that, I was juggling a job, managing a side business, and embarking on the dreadful dating process again.

It was a lot to handle, and I already felt drained.

LOVE LANGUAGES

I have forever been a hopeless romantic, yearning for the pure, simple pleasures that romance can bring: the sweet aroma of flowers, the handwritten love letters and notes, the thrill of surprise dates and weekend getaways, the little gifts, the joy of cooking dinner together, and the enchantment of candlelit evenings.

After my recent breakup, I set out to seek and savor these moments independently. With a newfound sense of abundance, I gave myself the type of treatment I had longed for by creating my own opportunities.

I dedicated my time to personal growth: reading, understanding my emotions, and uncovering my true needs. I realized that, above all else, I had the power to nourish and fulfill myself; I had to meet my own needs before expecting others to do so for me.

In moments of self-reflection, I grappled with questions of worthiness. What makes me deserving of good treatment? Do I have a clear understanding of my desires? Can I accept and embrace what I long for from a potential partner? Will I even recognize "my person" when they come along, and how will they make me feel?

I was beginning to heal my self-worth and embrace my true purpose. I was proud of myself and my progress.

I became interested in love languages, a concept popularized by Dr. Gary Chapman in his book *The 5 Love Languages: The Secret to Love that Lasts*.[2] According to Chapman, each person has a primary love language and also a preferred way of giving and receiving love. Love is an intricate and magnificent feeling that looks different for everyone, and love languages extend beyond romantic relationships; they also apply to friendships and family connections.

Particularly in intimate relationships, though, understanding and speaking your partner's love language can improve communication, emotional connection, and overall satisfaction in your relationship.[3]

Here's a deeper look into each love language.

Physical Touch emphasizes the power of physical contact and affectionate gestures. Actions such as holding hands, hugging, kissing, public displays of affection, and other forms of physical intimacy are essential for feeling loved and connected.

Words of Affirmation are for people who need verbal expressions of love, appreciation, and encouragement, such as compliments, kind words, and letters that acknowledge their worth, efforts, and achievements.

Acts of Service centers around actions that support your partner. Acts of Service include doing chores, running errands, preparing meals, or assisting with responsibilities since these actions demonstrate thoughtfulness, care, and a willingness to alleviate your partner's burdens or worries.

Quality Time emphasizes undivided attention and meaningful presence. It involves spending dedicated time together, engaging in activities that both partners enjoy, planning dates, and actively listening and communicating.

Gift-giving is for those who appreciate the thoughtfulness and effort behind tangible presents. It's not about materialism but rather the symbolic gesture of love. Meaningful gifts reflect understanding, attentiveness, and consideration for the recipient's desires and preferences.[4]

Understanding these love languages allowed me to uncover the missing pieces in my previous relationships and friendships, and it revealed how my need to receive love in a certain way shaped my experiences. We all express and perceive love differently, and that is what makes us unique.

While focusing on personal growth and introspection, I realized that falling in love vastly differs from what we often see on social media or in movies. It dawned on me that my feelings for Sam were potentially misguided since I truly adored him, but due to my naivety and lack of experience, I might not have understood what love was or felt like at that time. Without a reference point, I found it hard to grasp the true essence of genuine romantic feelings. Instead, I had been captivated by the idea of him and the potential we had together.

Perhaps my first encounter with what could be called "true" love didn't happen in my past relationships. I thought it was "true" at the time. This was tested through a monumental encounter with another person who imparted valuable lessons about my self-worth.

Let's jump into that roller coaster.

DARCY, PART 1: ROLLER COASTER

Just a few weeks in, I believed I had found "the one": Darcy.[5] I hoped that this person was my reward after learning so many hard lessons from a divorce and a failed relationship. I thought the third time would be the charm.

In the initial stages of our relationship, I shared with him all the insights and theories I had learned from my past, trying to ensure I wouldn't repeat old mistakes within our new union. I felt proud to have such self-awareness while also being attuned to Darcy's needs.

We had moments of joy together—Darcy would surprise me frequently with flowers, compose beautiful messages, and cook me delicious meals, and we generally spent lots of time together. It felt invigorating, as if we were headed in the right direction.

And then bam. A complete 180-degree turn, totally out of nowhere.

Sarah and I were snuggled up on the couch with my dogs when Darcy's text messages started taking a strange turn. Concerned, I gave him a call.

"Hey, is everything okay? Something seems off," I said, putting the call on speaker so Sarah could listen in.

"Yeah, everything's fine," Darcy replied.

"Are you sure? I can sense something's not right," I persisted.

"Well, I wasn't planning to do this over the phone, but I'm ending our relationship," he said.

Sarah and I exchanged stunned looks. My heart began to race. This was completely unexpected, especially considering that we had been making future plans with my friends just twenty-four hours earlier, while having dinner.

I sat there, holding the phone, my hands trembling, tears streaming down my face. I couldn't help but think, "Not again. Why does this keep happening to me?" Sarah put her hand on the blanket, gently applying a comforting and reassuring pressure to my feet.

Before ending the call, Darcy suggested meeting in person, and for some reason, I agreed. I suppose I was seeking some closure. However, when we met, he simply reiterated his words to my face, his demeanor cold as ice. And that was it. Closure remained elusive.

I had developed strong feelings for Darcy, and he seemed to reciprocate them, but I couldn't change the reality. I was upset and bewildered, but I refused to let despair consume me. I just saw it as another lesson that needed to be learned.

LIFE AT STAKE

I was fortunate to have incredible friends who distracted me after what happened with Darcy. We went hiking, and I focused on my physical fitness. Also at this time, my business was flourishing; I moved into my own home, established healthy boundaries with several people, and found some much-needed peace.

I felt deep gratitude and hope for the future. I was moving on.

One weekend, around three weeks after the breakup, Sarah and I went on a long hike, took a refreshing dip in a cold lake, and decided to have a sleepover to celebrate a contract I had secured. However, I began to feel a bit unwell, experiencing stomach flu-like symptoms but without a fever. Sarah playfully suggested that I take a pregnancy test to eliminate the possibility. We both chuckled since we were about to open a bottle of champagne, but I obliged and took the test.

Well, my laughter quickly subsided, and time seemed to stand still. The two lines were bright red.

After what felt like an eternity, I finally stepped out of the bathroom, looked at Sarah, and said, "It's positive."

She was comfortably nestled on the couch with my dogs and scrolling on her phone. At first, she laughed, not taking what I'd said seriously, but then her expression turned serious. "You're not joking, are you?" she said.

Sarah leaped from the couch, tossed her phone behind her, and rushed to the bathroom to see the result for herself. When she returned, she faced me and held her hands out in front of her as if trying to ward off an enraged dog or a charging bear. Then, wrapping me in a hug, she whispered, "Suzanna, breathe. Just breathe." All at once, my composure vanished, and a wave of panic overcame me.

My initial reaction was "I need to tell my parents! What will they think of me?" However, Sarah quickly dismissed that idea, saying that I could make my own decisions. She was right. Instead of thinking about my health, desires, and life, I had thought of my parents and how this would "impact" them—I needed to prioritize myself.

Suddenly, none of my previous problems mattered. The external noise had faded into silence, and I had entered a new reality. "Fear" did not even come close to describe the emotions coursing through my psyche.

Following Sarah's advice, I informed Darcy, and his reaction was one of shock and panic, too. We decided to meet for the first time since the breakup. Although I had moved on to some extent, I still had some lingering feelings for him.

Darcy expressed deep remorse, dropping down on his knees, apologizing, assuring me that he'd never intended to mistreat me and had contemplated reaching out to me himself. And I chose to believe him.

Following a series of tests, I was informed that my health was threatened, and I was hospitalized. Suddenly, before I could decide anything, I had to choose between two distressing outcomes: remain in my current state and develop further health complications or terminate the pregnancy and protect my health.

To make matters worse, the ongoing pandemic meant I had to face this ordeal without anyone by my side in the hospital.

I found myself alone and afraid.

As I lay in the sterile hospital room with its pristine white walls, I longed for my mother. Clutching myself tightly, I whispered, "Mama . . . Mama . . ." I wanted the presence of a nurturing maternal figure, to be embraced and comforted during this time of vulnerability and isolation. It felt as if I had regressed to my childhood, craving the solace that only a mother's love could provide. So, I became that motherly figure for myself.

Despite all my love for my parents and what I had come to

understand and accept about them, acknowledging that they had done their best with the knowledge they had, I still yearned for a level of support that I had only experienced in my imagination, and that realization shattered me completely. Tears streamed down my face until exhaustion enveloped me, and I finally fell asleep.

A few hours later, I awoke, disoriented, thinking about how Babyshka had been similarly alone during her hospitalization. I wrapped the blankets around myself, creating a small cocoon-like tent where I could hide, and I cried uncontrollably until I passed out again.

The healthcare professionals urged me to decide soon due to the impact on my well-being. I felt trapped and without any good options in front of me. The negatives far outweighed any potential positives and literally endangered my very life.

I had to prioritize my health, and so, with a heavy heart, I made a choice that I carry with me every day.

It deeply saddened me that this was how my first experience of motherhood was ending. But it opened my eyes to the many facets of this complex topic. I realized that countless women undergo similar ordeals and suffer in silence, carrying the weight of societal shame on them for the difficult decisions they must make. I believe it is crucial to address this issue openly. Because why should someone shoulder this heavy burden alone?

This event was one of the main catalysts for me to write this book—I wanted to extend an olive branch to people of all genders, assuring them that their choices are legitimate, whatever they may be, to promote peace and acceptance. More and more people are bravely speaking up about their experiences; I want to be another voice of strength. Each person has a unique story to tell, and sometimes, all we need to do is create a safe space where our voices can be heard.

By openly and transparently sharing my experiences, I hope to help others feel seen.

I understand this topic is deeply intertwined with religious and political ideologies, each with its own opinions and perspectives. I wholeheartedly respect everyone's paths and decisions in life. Every woman will encounter her own set of positive and negative moments concerning her body and experiences. In the face of such storms, we must summon our courage and embrace the strength within. We must also support one another with empathy and understanding.

It is important to acknowledge that partners also play a role, whether as part of a support system or as caregivers, and their emotions, perspectives, and experiences should not be disregarded or overlooked.

My intention with this book is to foster empathy, understanding, and compassion, ensuring that every voice is valued and heard, regardless of gender, background, or personal beliefs.

Since that pivotal moment, an invincible spirit has flourished within me. This decision enlightened me regarding life's delicate, transient, and valuable nature.

I now trust myself implicitly.

I hope you can see the recurring theme in this book: the power to shape your life lies solely in your hands. Only you can help yourself, no matter how challenging life gets.

DARCY, PART 2: COMPLETING THE CIRCLE

A few months after that life-altering event, when I had regained a semblance of a normal life, Darcy resurfaced and asked to meet with me. He said that he missed me and wished to reconcile, intending to approach the relationship more earnestly and thoroughly this time. It was as if Pandora's box had been reopened, stirring up a flurry of emotions. He spoke all the right words, appeared sorry for his past mistakes, and offered promises that aligned with my deepest desires, weaving a captivating fairy tale that felt impossible to resist. It became difficult not to entertain the idea, especially considering what we had already weathered together.

After the meeting, I discussed it with Sarah and a group of our girlfriends over a bottle of wine. I recounted every detail, eager for their perspectives and advice on what I should do.

"I'm not sure, Suzanna," Sarah said. "It sounds like a carefully crafted script to me. Why now? His timing seems quite self-centered. As you start to feel better and move forward, he reappears and pulls you back in. Maybe he genuinely misses you—I wouldn't be surprised if he does. But the whole situation appears too convenient. I'm having a hard time trusting it."

The other girls nodded, and one of them added, "When I met him, I didn't get the best vibe. And the way he resurfaced was out of the blue. Is this really what you want?"

Their doubts echoed my own. "Yeah, I'm at a loss, too," I confessed. "It does seem random, but isn't that just life? Part of me will always wonder if I don't give it a shot . . . you know, what if things actually work out this time? What if all of this was somehow meant to happen?" I knew I sounded a little naive.

Sarah just crossed her arms and rolled her eyes. Still, she and my other friends had my back. "Suz, you'll ultimately make the right choice, and we'll stand by you no matter what. Just think hard about it," Sarah said. "Personally, if I were in your shoes, I'd run in the other direction and cut my losses."

"Yeah, I'd probably do the same," another friend said while sipping her wine.

But I was stubborn.

Despite the advice of my closest friends, I still decided to give him a second chance, hoping for the best. I couldn't stand the idea of leaving that relationship unexplored. The fear of the unknown, the lingering "what if," kept me bound to him. In hindsight, the girls were right; I should have run in the opposite direction, but I didn't.

The first month we reunited was delightful; we took a couple of trips and comfortably established ourselves together. Yet, as time passed, the initial euphoria quickly faded.

I realized I had compromised my core values by giving this

union a second chance. I rapidly lost touch with my true self, dimming my energy and light because he found it overpowering.

This led me to isolate myself, worrying my friends, who wondered why I had become withdrawn. I attempted to fit into the narrow confines Darcy had set for me, molding myself into what he desired, hoping to receive his love and approval. Darcy deemed anything outside those confines "embarrassing" and saw it as a threat to his "perfect reputation." The dynamic we created left no room for my energy. Hence, I channeled everything I had into my business to fill the void in my personal life.

This entire experience was the final, if not main, lesson that taught me the importance of self-respect and staying true to myself, learning to trust my intuition, and gracefully departing from something that no longer served me.

I had reached a point of complete exhaustion. I wasn't angry or upset, just done. All I wanted was to protect myself and salvage the remnants of my peace.

It is often unwise to step into the same river twice, especially when not enough time has passed. People do not typically undergo significant transformations so quickly. Change requires time, introspection, and deliberate efforts.

I now believe that what drew me back to this relationship was what experts call a trauma bond.

A trauma bond is a complex psychological phenomenon that occurs when an individual forms an intense emotional attachment to someone who has caused them emotional pain or trauma or with whom they went through a life-altering experience. It often arises in situations characterized by a cycle of highs and lows, manipulation, and a distorted sense of love and loyalty.[6]

REFLECTIONS
ON IDENTIFYING A TRAUMA BOND

Identifying whether you are caught in a trauma bond can be challenging, as it often involves conflicting emotions and blurred boundaries. However, there are some common signs to observe:

- Your relationship may go through extreme moments of intense closeness, affection, and passion and periods of conflict, emotional distance, or even abuse.
- You may be seeking and feeling reliant on their validation and approval as a source of self-worth.
- You may make excuses for the other person's actions, blame yourself, or minimize their negative impact on your life.
- The person you are bonded to may subtly or overtly discourage you from maintaining connections with friends, family, or other sources of support.
- Despite the pain and toxicity, you may have an intense fear of leaving the relationship, driven by the belief that no one else would understand or accept you in the same way.[7]

Recognizing these signs is an important step toward breaking free from a trauma bond. Seek support from trusted friends, family, and/or professionals who can guide, validate, and help as you navigate the process.

On a random afternoon, Darcy ended our relationship. Once more. It had become a pattern, and deep down, I confess, a part of me had sensed this coming.

I had been thinking of doing it myself, actually.

Instead of navigating the complexities of our connection with caution and introspection, I had recklessly jumped into their depths. Why did I crave Darcy's validation so desperately? Perhaps it was the siren call of the "what if" or the insidious grip of a trauma bond laced tightly around my wounded heart, whispering false promises of comfort and redemption.

I now consider the end of my time with Darcy my graduation from the halls of hell.

I was right after all; the third time was the charm. Getting back together and breaking up again completed the circle of lessons I needed to learn, allowing me to break free. After so much chaos, I finally experienced my *forelsket*. I irreversibly fell in love with myself, who I was, and how I was.

I realized that I could not build a home in someone else, that I had to trust myself more, and that I would never allow anyone else to hurt me the same way again.

Understanding all of that is what enabled my ultimate transformation.

I found peace.

7

~~SERENDIPITY:~~ EMBRACING THE RHYTHM OF LIFE

["Serendipity": noun / ˌser-ən-ˈdi-pə-tē/]
The faculty or phenomenon of finding valuable or agreeable things not sought for.[1]

AFTER THREE UNSUCCESSFUL ATTEMPTS, I took a break from relationships. I dedicated the time to absorb all the life lessons and assume responsibility for my roles and actions within the relationships, and it became essential for me to focus on healing and implementing the lessons into my daily life.

With this newfound perspective, I traveled across Europe, indulging in all the experiences I had always yearned for. I visited the countries that had captivated my imagination, enjoyed their food, and spent time with friends who made me feel complete. This adventure was a gift to myself for all my personal growth.

Throughout my travels, I continued to write this book, finding inspiration in the diverse landscapes. I was living my *Eat, Pray, Love* moment.[2]

Vulnerably sharing my story through this book, with the mission to help, was uncharted territory for me, and I felt intense fear of how it would be received and perceived. Yet, my intuition consistently whispered to me with assurances that the "it" I had within me had guided me right to this moment. I believe that the experiences I've gained revealed my purpose—to extend a supporting hand to others, empowering them to embark on their own transformative journeys and embrace life's boundless potential.

It wasn't about me anymore.

I know now that having ultimate control over one's future is an illusion. While we can't predict what life will throw at us, we do hold the power to choose how we respond to the challenges it presents. Our past experiences equip us to face future obstacles, and though we may encounter new challenges, our ability to adapt and grow remains a constant source of empowerment.

Even though many things are out of our control, we still have the power to keep a positive mindset and manifest. Manifestation is the process of bringing your desires and intentions into reality through positive thinking, focused thought, belief, and action.[3] It is based on the principle that our thoughts and emotions can shape our external circumstances. By aligning our mindset, beliefs, and actions with what we want to achieve or attract, we can manifest positive outcomes and experiences.

While I recognize that the idea of manifestation may not resonate with everyone, I can attest to its effectiveness in my life. Therefore, I want to introduce this concept from my lens, and offer you resources to help you incorporate it into your life if you wish to.

REFLECTIONS
ON MANIFESTATION

I have followed and developed the steps below over a decade of trial and error practicing manifestation.

> **Clarify** what you truly want to manifest. Simply ask yourself, "What do I want?" Be specific and detailed about your intentions. Write them down in a journal or create a dream board to visually represent your goals. I always categorize my manifestations into these categories:
>
> - Career aspirations
> - Passion projects
> - Milestones
> - Possessions (house, car, etc.)
> - Financial gains (long and short term)
> - Love and relationships
> - Travel destinations
> - Lifestyle
>
> It truly can be anything that you dream of. However, keeping your goals "realistic" and "attainable" when you are starting is key, as consistency plays a big role in this practice.

Your path to manifestation is not always straightforward, but it's essential to subconsciously direct your energy toward it. So, during moments of low inspiration and when your goals seem distant, focus on general thoughts about your objectives. On the other hand, when you feel more inspired and closer to reaching a goal, be more specific in your manifestations.

Create a mental image of yourself already living your desired outcome. Engage all your senses to make the visualization vivid and immersive. Feel the emotions associated with achieving your goals, allowing yourself to experience joy, gratitude, and fulfillment as if they have already happened.[4]

Cultivate credence in your ability to manifest your desires. Release any doubts, limiting beliefs, or resistance that might hinder your progress. Trust in the process and that everything is working in your favor, even when you do not see it immediately—and sometimes that's the hardest part.

Break down your goals into actionable steps and pursue them with dedication and intention. Manifestation requires more than just wishful thinking.

Nurture an outlook of gratitude for what you already have and the manifestations that are on their way. Gratitude amplifies positive energy and aligns you with abundance. Sometimes, we fail to recognize that we are experiencing what we previously worked to manifest. Gratitude puts this into perspective for us.

Remember that manifestation is a process, and life's timing may not always align with your expectations. Trust in divine timing and have patience. Stay committed to your intentions while remaining open to the possibilities and lessons that come your way.

This is the difficult part: letting go of control. I was only able to achieve that for the first time when I hit rock bottom. However, once I understood what it felt like, I was able to enter a state of trust in a healthier manner.

It is important to note that manifestation is not a magic solution and does not guarantee instant results. It requires consistent practice, a positive mindset, and aligned action over time. By incorporating manifestation techniques into your daily life and maintaining a positive and proactive approach, you can harness the power of manifestation to create the life you desire.

MANIFESTING MICHAEL

Despite my self-sufficiency and purpose, around half a year after the breakup, I decided to put the energy into manifesting my future life and partner so that I could receive it all when the time was right. I returned to the practice of writing my intentions and desires.

Through this intentional and thoughtful approach, I aimed to attract a partner who would complement me and contribute positively to my life. I didn't put any pressure on it. I simply felt proud that I was gradually preparing to venture into the realm of companionship once more.

REFLECTIONS
ON MANIFESTING A COMPATIBLE PARTNER

I strongly recommend those of you who are seeking a partner to give this exercise a try, as it can genuinely assist you in aligning your thoughts and reflecting on what you are looking for.

- Outline the qualities, values, and characteristics you desire in a partner, focusing on the person's essence and the traits that complement your own. List qualities important to you in a partner, such as kindness, humor, ambition, or empathy.
- Reflect on the stage in your life when you envision meeting this partner.
- Explore the settings or circumstances in which your paths might cross.
- Analyze the emotions and experiences you desire in a relationship to create a deep connection and sense of fulfillment.
- Identify nonnegotiable values and boundaries, ensuring alignment with your personal beliefs and goals.

You know that saying "Sometimes you find what you're looking for when you least expect it"? I used to be skeptical about it until it happened to me. *One Failure at a Time* was initially intended to explore only the difficult lessons life teaches us, hence the title. But this book has an unexpected ending, which I believe is a reward for embracing my true purpose. It can also demonstrate that despite hardships, there is potentially a light at the end of the tunnel. So, I decided to share this new stage of my life with you.

I wasn't actively seeking a relationship or hoping to meet someone anytime soon. In fact, I was quite content focusing on my own happiness and life. However, by chance, I crossed paths with someone who would have a lasting impact on my reality from day one—Michael.[5]

Michael and I had several informal encounters before we were officially introduced at an international work event. Unbeknownst to us, a professional colleague of ours was secretly playing matchmaker, orchestrating our connection behind the scenes.

Michael became my impromptu chaperone during the event—our matchmaker colleague ensured it. I became his responsibility, and due to my busy schedule, we rushed between different speaking engagements and events.

This was also Michael's initial exposure to who I was. He witnessed my professional competence and intensity while catching a glimpse of the quieter, more reserved side of me behind the scenes.

Between meetings, after spending extensive time together, Michael and I found ourselves sharing a coffee break.

"I feel like I'm witnessing something truly unique," he casually said, reaching for his coffee.

I looked at him, a blend of curiosity and amusement in my expression, raising an eyebrow to signal my puzzlement at his statement.

He smiled. "You're an unstoppable force on stage and in business, yet in between, you're gentle and soft-spoken. That combination and balance is quite rare."

I found his observations intriguing, as it was a perspective I hadn't encountered before. He simultaneously appreciated my robust masculine energy and soft feminine side.

"Thank you for saying that, Michael," I muttered, my tone tinged with shyness.

I felt seen.

From that moment on, I began to see him in a new light. It was a special moment.

As the sun set on the first eventful day, we decided to extend the evening. We went out for drinks and even found ourselves attending another conference after-party that occurred simultaneously. This conference was on the subject of sprinklers—yes, sprinklers. The enthusiasm with which the attendees discussed these mundane devices fascinated us. It was a refreshing change from the serious issues we usually dealt with in our professional lives. We joined in the discussions with the irrigation professionals, shared laughs and cocktails, and enjoyed cigars.

Being around Michael felt effortless; our shared sense of humor made joking around a breeze. As professionals in the same field, we conversed in a language unique to our industry, and the familiarity was rejuvenating.

The conference-related festivities winded down, but we didn't want the night to end. My sudden craving for a burger at 4:00 a.m. became a shared adventure. I offered to go alone, but Michael insisted on accompanying me. And so off we went into the early morning darkness in pursuit of a burger. Our expedition took over an hour, leading us through quiet streets as we navigated our way to satiate my hunger.

Sitting on the floor of my hotel room, the two of us, famished and exhausted, shared stories, glee, and those coveted burgers. Time seemed to stretch and bend as we lost ourselves in conversation, completely unaware of the advancing hours. With the morning sun beginning to illuminate the world outside, we realized that dawn was upon us, and it was time to prepare for the day's conference activities.

Sleep had eluded us that night, yet the spark of connection and the excitement propelled us forward. Throughout the conference, our bond grew, and our conversations continued to flow effortlessly.

From that moment on, we became inseparable.

Michael and I were like kindred spirits who had been separated. We shared similar childhoods, heritage, immigration stories, and life experiences.

Meeting him felt like a jolt running through me, and as time passed, we found ourselves in a healthy relationship built on mutual respect and open communication.

From the start, we naturally dove into deep conversations, addressing all topics honestly and without sugarcoating anything so that we could understand our pasts, love languages, needs, wants, attachments, and conflict styles. We discussed our vulnerabilities and triggers, ensuring we never crossed lines that could harm our relationship. If we did encounter any issues, we faced them together and immediately tried to resolve them. Michael consistently reassured me, saying, "I am here for you, no matter what. I am not leaving your side." He had learned to navigate me, as I, him, which I now know is one of the most crucial aspects of a committed relationship and partnership. Without that foundation, what's the point of being together?

We genuinely wanted to understand each other and make things work, and our desires aligned so wholly that it felt almost surreal.

Being with Michael made me realize how much I had settled in the past.

Not everyone gets the chance to experience this type of "spark" and love—I believe that only the ones who do the introspective work on themselves might one day experience this euphoria. Of course, it all comes down to the context and circumstances in the grand scheme of things. We can never be sure or make accurate predictions about the outcome or magnitude of anything.

We can just try our best.

This is the very motivation behind my book—to share what I've discovered, enabling you to engage with your emotions and potentially find the same sense of liberation I have achieved through my trials.

DEVELOPING A SECURE ATTACHMENT

I find that understanding the basics of how we get attached is necessary for a healthy relationship. According to British psychologist, psychiatrist, and psychoanalyst John Bowlby and American-Canadian psychologist Mary Ainsworth, attachment styles are fundamental patterns of how individuals relate and connect to others. There are several attachment styles, and much research has been conducted on this topic, especially concerning childhood relationships.[6] Over the years, I've had my own experiences regarding attachment styles. Here are the three styles that have stood out to me as an adult in my relationships.

Individuals with an **insecure attachment** style often struggle with feelings of anxiety and uncertainty in relationships. They may constantly need reassurance and validation from their partners, fearing abandonment and rejection. People with insecure attachment might also exhibit clingy behaviors, struggle with trust, and have difficulty expressing their needs effectively.[7]

Those with a **secure attachment** style tend to have healthy, balanced relationships. Individuals with secure attachments feel comfortable with both intimacy and independence. They have strong self-worth and can form deep connections with others while maintaining autonomy. They trust their partners and believe in their own ability to navigate relationship challenges.[8]

The **avoidant attachment** style is characterized by a strong desire for independence and self-reliance. They tend to value their freedom and personal space, often avoiding emotional intimacy and becoming uncomfortable with too much closeness. People with an avoidant attachment style may struggle with commitment, suppress emotions, and maintain emotional distance in relationships.[9]

It's important to note that attachment styles can evolve or blend over time as individuals gain self-awareness and engage in therapeutic interventions. Developing a secure attachment style is an achievable goal, even for those who have experienced insecure or avoidant attachment patterns in the past. Therapy, self-reflection, and building emotional resilience can be valuable tools in this process, helping you create more secure and satisfying relationships and connections.[10]

BUILDING OUR BENCH

Effective communication is not just about expressing our feelings and thoughts; it's about truly understanding one another. We foster a deeper connection with our partners by actively listening and by recognizing the underlying emotions and motivations behind their words and actions.

Michael is a bit old-school and traditional, a value that was unfortunately suppressed in his past relationships. He harbored a strong desire for a family and children; however, his previous connections did not prioritize those aspirations, which led him to question whether these dreams were meant for him.

Our shared histories became catalysts for growth and resilience in our relationship. Just as I had, Michael took the time to absorb and reflect on the lessons each experience had taught him. He, too, had been in three significant relationships before crossing paths with me. In hindsight, he recognized that he should have distanced himself from those relationships well before they eventually deteriorated. Yet, the allure of comfort and the persistent fear of the "what if" significantly affected how long he stayed.

It was largely through our conversations that Michael discovered what was missing in his previous relationships. His determination to avoid repeating his mistakes and preserve our union's peace and love reaffirmed my approach of laying everything on the table at the beginning and working together to create a strong foundation.

Michael and I often compare relationships to constructing a bench, a process that requires careful planning and execution. Just as a sturdy bench requires a strong foundation, relationships thrive when we lay down solid groundwork. Together, we must establish a clear vision and set goals and expectations. Understanding each other's needs and desires forms the basis of a sturdy and fulfilling connection.

We carefully choose the materials that best suit our needs as we construct a bench. Likewise, we must identify the essential elements that create strength and longevity in relationships. Love, trust, communication, and respect become the building blocks for creating something beautiful and enduring.

And constructing a bench doesn't end with its assembly. We must refine its appearance, maintain it, and protect it from environmental factors. Similarly, relationships require nurturing and regular maintenance; we must address any issues that arise and put effort into keeping the love and connection alive.

Relationships can suffer cracks just like a bench may experience wear and tear. But how we handle these damages defines the strength of our commitment. Like a rough patch in a relationship, a wobble or chipped paint on a bench presents an opportunity for growth and adaptation. Instead of dismissing the bench or the relationship as imperfect, we can invest our time and energy into improving it, making it the best version possible—as long as the foundation is still intact.

MASCULINE AND FEMININE UNITED

As we were chatting about the bench, Michael shared that he hadn't experienced the nurturing he needed early in his life from his parents, nor had he found a partner who listened to and honored what mattered most to him—someone who understood his values and saw him for who he was.

After his three attempts at love, Michael embraced his true self, cultural background, and traditional values, establishing a clear life path for him and strengthening his masculinity. As he shared this with me, I was also undergoing my own transformation by awakening elements of my femininity that had been bottled up before. We were on similar trajectories to embrace our authenticity.

As I mentioned in previous chapters, I faced challenges with past partners due to the dynamics within the relationship, often finding myself predominantly in a masculine energy state. However, Michael's support and the safe space he provided allowed me to begin embracing my feminine essence for the first time in my life. This opened a new pathway of ease and contentment within me, benefiting both of us.

Our relationship is not perfect, but we do make the effort to work at it every day.

Mental health and establishing boundaries were never given priority in Michael's past experiences and relationships, so we also explored these topics together. We built our foundation through transparency, daily reassurances, and intentional actions. This foundation has transformed my relationship dreams into reality and guided me toward peace in my personal life.

Michael says the best part of our relationship is the sensation of "coming home" since, amid the chaos of the outside world, the peacefulness between us is a tranquil oasis.

Well, the feeling was certainly mutual.

He often goes back to the moment we met, and even though we have now been together for a while, he still likes to recall that event. "Right from the start, what impressed me was your openness in sharing your fears, mistakes, past experiences, and candid emotions. You communicated them all, whether they brought you hurt, betrayal, happiness, or insecurity. That part of you greatly contributed to the bond we formed. While some might view it as a weakness, I saw it as a testament to your honesty, strength, and resilience."

He continued. "Your romantic side surfaced early in our relationship, too—the adorable good morning and good night texts, the expressive emojis, the gratitude you expressed, and your enthusiasm for planning dates. Your unabashed romantic nature was something I found endearing and admired—you embraced it so easily, so wholeheartedly."

There are moments when I struggle to accept everything Michael says about me, as being perceived in this way was a foreign concept to me for nearly three decades. His openness, however, has been a valuable contribution to my healing process.

HEALTHY CONFLICT RESOLUTION

However, even the healthiest relationships have differences and can include conflict. Michael smiled as he recalled, "We thoroughly explored our perspectives on life, expectations, partnership, and connection, including discussions about marriage and children. Our cultural backgrounds aligned, as did our personalities. Yet, we had our differences. For instance, you had a meticulous approach to daily life, whereas I was more calculated in my professional sphere but laid back in my personal life."

I knew just what he was referring to. While we were separated early in our relationship due to my international travels, I took the initiative to plan activities for when we finally could meet. Excitedly, I told him, "I'll send you calendar invites for our planned dates, along with detailed descriptions and color-coded categories for each activity," only to be met with shocked silence.

Michael eventually voiced his confusion, saying, "What do you mean 'send calendar invites' for our dates? That's a bit unusual."

His response caught me off guard, and I felt my heart race.

"We don't need such structured planning," he continued, surprised that the topic had even arisen. "We know we'll meet, and we can go with the flow."

But I stood firm. "Michael, there's value in this approach," I said. "I'm a businesswoman, and this structure ensures I allocate my time efficiently, giving my all to each task. This method suits me at this stage of my life; I can't entirely rely on spontaneity."

This marked the first time I asserted my true self in a new relationship—a personal milestone—and it was our first minor divergence in the few months we'd been together. While differences inevitably arose from our personalities, experiences, triggers, and lifestyles, he consistently supported my self-expression.

Michael reassured me that he didn't view my need for structure negatively; it simply surprised him because it differed from his approach and that of past partners. He also acknowledged that the infancy of our relationship factored into his response. But my high-performance mindset resonated with him, prompting him to adopt aspects of my structured approach into his personal life.

He said, "As I pieced together information about you, your upbringing, and your past relationships, I realized the importance of precision and organization in your life. I recognized the need to meet you on that level to facilitate personal growth."

The beauty of this resolution lies in our open communication. We discussed the significance of our actions, feelings, and needs and incorporated these insights into our relationship. It was the first time I felt safe enough to engage in such a dialogue with a partner—devoid of judgment, argument, or harmful resistance.

I share this with you so you can discover your own path to healthy conflict resolution. Understanding your and your partner's conflict styles is crucial for cultivating a healthy relationship.

Conflict is inevitable in human interaction, and people adopt different styles to manage it. These conflict styles represent the habitual patterns of behavior that individuals exhibit when confronted with disagreement or discord. Grasping these different styles can provide insights into how individuals navigate conflicts and interact in challenging situations.

Here are the five conflict styles by Kenneth Thomas and Ralph Kilmann in *Thomas-Kilmann Conflict Mode Instrument*:[11]

> **Collaborative Style** is when individuals express their needs, concerns, and opinions while actively listening to others. They strive for a win-win outcome by seeking collaborative solutions that address the interests of all parties involved. This style promotes open communication, mutual respect, and constructive problem-solving.

Avoidant Style is when individuals shy away from confrontation and prefer to minimize conflicts altogether. They may withdraw from a situation, ignore the issue, or postpone discussions. While this style can temporarily reduce tension, it may hinder the resolution of underlying problems and lead to unresolved conflicts.

Accommodating Style involves prioritizing the needs and desires of others over one's own. Individuals with this style are inclined to compromise or give in to maintain harmony in the relationship.

Competitive Style is when individuals assert their interests and goals above all else. They often adopt a win-lose mentality, seeking to maximize their benefits while disregarding the concerns and needs of others.

Compromising Style involves seeking a common ground where both parties can make concessions and reach a mutually acceptable solution. Individuals expressing this style are willing to concede certain aspects of their position to achieve a balanced outcome.[12]

It is important to note that conflict styles are not fixed or rigid; individuals can employ different styles depending on the situation, their personal preferences, and the dynamics with others involved. Developing self-awareness and understanding the various conflict styles can facilitate more effective communication and collaboration.[13]

My counselor once told me, "When you find yourself upset with your partner over something they may have done, it is better to express that 'a part of me is upset with you' rather than simply stating 'I am upset with you.'" This distinction allows for a more nuanced and compassionate approach to addressing conflicts. By acknowledging that only a part of us is upset, we communicate that our love and commitment to our partner remain intact. Simultaneously, we address the specific action or behavior that caused the distress, fostering open dialogue and understanding.[14]

I believe that my counselor's advice is one of the most crucial things to remember when communicating your needs to your partner to avoid miscommunication and emotional neglect. You are emphasizing that a specific part of you needs fulfillment and attention. If it is your entire being that is unfulfilled, that may indicate a whole other problem that needs to be addressed.

This approach to conflict resolution recognizes that our emotions can be multifaceted. By separating our emotions into parts, we can communicate with empathy and compassion while addressing specific issues within our relationships. It nurtures a safe and supportive environment for both partners to express themselves and work through challenges together.

Michael came into my life as a graduation gift and a surprise that would guide me into the pages of my next chapter in life. With his arrival, I felt inspired, like the ink of a pen longing to create a love story.

When I was manifesting and reflecting on my current needs in this phase of my life, I knew I wanted the opportunity to build a family and have children in a healthy and loving relationship, which has become a reality with Michael. I was able to share every aspect of my past in a supportive environment; this enabled me to expand my wings and soar.

He is a vision that found its way to me sooner than I ever anticipated.

I manifested Michael.

CONCLUSION

NAVĪNA ĀTMAN: UNEARTHING INNER EVOLUTION

["Navīna Ātman": noun]
Renewed self: an evolution within oneself, a process of inner transformation that leads to a renewed sense of identity and purpose.[1]

SO WHERE DO YOU GO from here?

Within these pages, you followed the winding narrative that led me to several realizations.

This book aimed to share some of my life experiences and research to show you that having an unfiltered and imperfect life is not only acceptable but also valuable.

My ultimate goal was for individuals at any point in their lives to see that a single decision, within or outside their control, can be the key to attaining or redirecting to the life they authentically desire.

I also wanted to demonstrate that life does not follow a linear path; it is laced with moments of extraordinary joy and intense despair.

At the beginning of this book, you encountered a version of me who boldly ventured into her twenties armed with a meticulously crafted checklist and dutifully ticking off each item. Yet, despite the appearance of success, a deep discontentment lurked within. I had deviated from authenticity for the sake of external validation.

When I began to question my reality, I saw how my early childhood experiences helped me achieve great things but prevented me from truly understanding myself. Gradually, I learned to place self-care and self-worth at the forefront of my decision-making, cultivating genuine self-love and resilience in the face of life's challenges. Living according to someone else's expectations can eventually lead us to overlook unexplored opportunities, which may slowly result in regret and resentment. Therefore, developing the ability to prioritize your own fulfillment over the fear of disappointing others is essential to lead an authentic and peaceful life. Once you reach that level of inner peace, protect it at all costs because only you know what it took to get there.

A pearl of wisdom is captured in a Russian proverb: "Once burned by milk, you will blow on cold water." This simple phrase encapsulates the lessons I learned from my past experiences, which taught me to be more vigilant and discerning as I navigated new situations. I had many opportunities to surrender and abandon my efforts when facing challenges. My progress could have ended at any of those moments if I chose to quit, but I kept growing. I chose to. Everything is a choice. Our mindset is what separates us from the rest. The so-called "failure" could have gotten the best of me at any time. It took nearly three decades of continual personal growth for me to reach this point, but it was well worth it. Don't you think? Now, I can arm you with a survival guide forged from these hard-earned lessons.

I am grateful to my parents, whom I hold dear, who worked tirelessly to raise my sister and me and provide opportunities that enabled us to flourish. Their methodology wasn't perfect, but every encounter shaped me. All that happened in the past is now forgiven; I've fully embraced my parents for who they are, and I profoundly appreciate their sacrifices.

All the people who entered my life and then departed, leaving behind their teachings, also paved the way for the writing of this book. It feels extraordinary to look back at something and see it from a perspective of gratitude and peace. Each moment has been a stepping stone toward sharing my knowledge and insights with you.

All my experiences have empowered me to stand as an advocate for humanity. My ultimate desire is for people to uncover the wisdom within themselves that can illuminate their paths forward.

And so, I ask you: What are you prepared to do to forgive, heal, and ultimately liberate yourself from everything that caused and is causing you inner turmoil?

I hope this book has answered any questions you might've had or even helped you discover any obstacles that have stagnated your evolution. Or perhaps it just reinforced the idea that whatever you are going through right now is okay or will be okay. One day, you might wake up and look back on this period of your life and be so proud that you did not give up despite the adversities.

My father, whose journey has also come full circle, is now a university professor. These days, when he steps into the classroom to teach, he often asks his students a question that might seem unusual: "Are you struggling?"

When they reply with a hesitant yes, he responds with genuine delight and a smile, saying, "I am so happy for you. The fact that you're facing and overcoming challenges means you're actively engaging and growing."

And he is right. My father always told my sister and me that venturing beyond your comfort zone and embracing what others deem "risky" often comes with unique rewards. Through these courageous acts, you can tap into your true potential and achieve personal and spiritual growth. While challenges may arise, the resilience and skills you acquire through these experiences can be transformative, leading to a greater understanding of yourself and the world.

Always remember that it is never too late for a new beginning or to bring closure to a chapter in your life. To truly change, you must challenge your preconceived notions, reevaluate your core beliefs, and reassess how you perceive personal and professional triumphs and setbacks. Time will keep going, whether you do something or not. It does not stop for anyone; it is merciless. So, it is your choice, months or years from now. Will you be looking back at excuses or progress?

You hold the reins to your own life, dear reader. You craft the narrative, choose the plot twists, and decide which characters will inhabit your story. Like a skilled author, you hold the pen that writes your future. Moreover, you set the standards for how you want to be treated, and you teach others how to interact with you.

May you embark on the journey of self-discovery, engage in

inner work, experience healing, and ultimately blossom into the best version of yourself.

You deserve it.

ACKNOWLEDGMENTS

Writing this book was a challenge, as it delves deep into personal territories, leaving me feeling vulnerable. The realization that it's now completed and out in the world continues to astonish me. This project stands as one of the most beautiful endeavors I've ever attempted, demanding a year and a half of relentless dedication, seven months abroad in Europe, a significant financial investment, the support of my partner, encouragement from twelve loyal friends, guidance from four lawyers, and the backing of an incredible online community. This book is also the culmination of the first three decades of my life. It's a humbling reminder of how I have thrived and survived.

The decision to take the self-publishing route was intentional; I felt strongly that this was my story to share—on my own terms. Moreover, I wanted to intimately understand the intricacies of the publishing process to pave the way for future works.

As this book was edited, I embarked on a challenging journey pursuing a PhD while managing a full-time business. This phase involved late nights for months, eighteen-hour workdays, countless emails, tears, and moments of loneliness and doubt that nearly convinced me to cease the entire process. The fear of how my story would be interpreted loomed large, yet the "it" inside me pushed me forward—to share my experiences with the hope of offering solace or deeper self-understanding to others.

In unexpected ways, writing this book became a therapeutic outlet, granting me a voice. What is funny is that even after I believed I had healed most aspects within me, this process unearthed additional lingering elements embedded in my heart—an acknowledgment that this is an ongoing, lifelong process I've come to accept and love.

To those who stood by me during moments of doubt—professionals who shared their expertise and friends who empathized with my struggles—I am profoundly grateful to you. Your encouragement and donated time propelled me forward during moments when I questioned my ability to continue.

To you, the reader, my sincere thanks for investing your time in reading this book. Your trust and belief in my story is invaluable. I hope what I've learned adds value to your life. We just have to keep moving forward one step at a time!

We've got this!

NOTES

NOTES

INTRODUCTION

1. Merriam-Webster. (n.d.). Enigmatic. In *Merriam-Webster.com dictionary*. Retrieved August 18, 2023, from https://www.merriam-webster.com/dictionary/enigmatic
2. While this quote is often attributed to Brené Brown, the exact source is unknown.
3. Obama, M. (2018). *Becoming*. Crown Publishing Group.
4. A source of general inspiration for this book is Manson, M. (2016). *The subtle art of not giving a f*ck: A counterintuitive approach to living a good life*. Harper.
5. Carnegie, D. (1970). *How to enjoy your life and your job: Selections from how to win friends and influence people, and how to stop worrying and start living*. Simon & Schuster.
6. Manson, M. (2016). *The subtle art of not giving a f*ck: A counterintuitive approach to living a good life*. Harper.
7. Manson, M. (2016). *The subtle art of not giving a f*ck: A counterintuitive approach to living a good life*. Harper.

CHAPTER 1

1. Finlandia University. (n.d.). *Our history & heritage*. Retrieved July 26, 2022, from https://www.finlandia.edu/about/heritage/.
2. Tyyskä, V. (2007). *Immigrant families in sociology*. In J. E. Lansford, K. Deater-Deckard, & M. H. Bornstein (Eds.), *Immigrant families in contemporary society* (pp. 83–99). The Guilford Press.
3. Fleck, J. R., & Fleck, D. T. (2013). The immigrant family: Parent-child dilemmas and therapy considerations. *American International Journal of Contemporary Research*, 3(8), 13–17. https://aijcrnet.com/journals/Vol_3_No_8_August_2013/2.pdf
4. Muccino, G. (Director). (2006). *The pursuit of happyness* [Film]. Columbia Pictures.
5. Fleming N. D. (2001). *Teaching and learning styles: VARK strategies*. Neil D Fleming.
6. Fleming N. D. (2001). *Teaching and learning styles: VARK strategies*. Neil D Fleming.
7. Gardner, H. (2011). *Frames of mind: The theory of multiple intelligences*. Basic Books.
8. Gardner, H. (2011). *Frames of mind: The theory of multiple intelligences*. Basic Books.

9. Gardner, H. (2011). *Frames of mind: The theory of multiple intelligences.* Basic Books.
10. Gardner, H. (2011). *Frames of mind: The theory of multiple intelligences.* Basic Books.
11. Van der Kolk, B. (2015). *The body keeps the score: Brain, mind, and body in the healing of trauma.* Penguin Books.
12. Van der Kolk, B. (2015). *The body keeps the score: Brain, mind, and body in the healing of trauma.* Penguin Books.
13. Edwards, V.J., Holden, G.W., Felitti, V.J., & Anda, R.F. (2003). Relationship between multiple forms of childhood maltreatment and adult mental health in community respondents: results from the adverse childhood experiences study. American Journal of Psychiatry, 160(8), 1453-60. https://doi.org/10.1176/appi.ajp.160.8.1453
14. Edwards, V.J., Holden, G.W., Felitti, V.J., & Anda, R.F. (2003). Relationship between multiple forms of childhood maltreatment and adult mental health in community respondents: results from the adverse childhood experiences study. American Journal of Psychiatry, 160(8), 1453-60. https://doi.org/10.1176/appi.ajp.160.8.1453
15. Leeb R. T., Paulozzi L. J., Melanson C., Simon T. R., and Arias I. (2008). *Child maltreatment surveillance: Uniform definitions for public health and recommended data elements.* National Center for Injury Prevention and Control (U.S.). https://hdl.loc.gov/loc.gdc/gdcebookspublic.2023692262
16. Leeb R. T., Paulozzi L. J., Melanson C., Simon T. R., and Arias I. (2008). *Child maltreatment surveillance: Uniform definitions for public health and recommended data elements.* National Center for Injury Prevention and Control (U.S.). https://hdl.loc.gov/loc.gdc/gdcebookspublic.2023692262
17. Gibson, L. C. (2022). *Adult children of emotionally immature parents: How to heal from distant, rejecting, or self-involved parents.* New Harbinger Publications, Inc.
18. Gibson, L. C. (2022). *Adult children of emotionally immature parents: How to heal from distant, rejecting, or self-involved parents.* New Harbinger Publications, Inc.
19. Shapiro, F. (2017). *Eye movement desensitization and reprocessing (EMDR) therapy: Basic principles, protocols, and procedures.* (3rd ed.). Guilford Press.
20. Goleman, D. (2005). *Emotional intelligence: Why it can matter more than IQ* (Revised Edition). Bantam Books.
21. Goleman, D. (2005). *Emotional intelligence: Why it can matter more than IQ* (Revised Edition). Bantam Books.
22. Webb, J., & Musello, C. (2012). *Running on empty: Overcome your childhood emotional neglect.* Morgan James Publishing.
23. Durvasula, R. (2015). *Should I stay or should I go: Surviving a relationship with a narcissist.* Post Hill Press.
24. Durvasula, R. (2015). *Should I stay or should I go: Surviving a relationship with a narcissist.* Post Hill Press.
25. Durvasula, R. (2015). *Should I stay or should I go: Surviving a relationship with a narcissist.* Post Hill Press.
26. March, E., Kay, C., Dinić, B., Wagstaff, D., Grabovac, B., & Jonason, P. (2023). "It's all in your head": Personality traits and gaslighting tactics in intimate

relationships. *Journal of Family Violence*, 1–10. https://doi.org/10.1007/s10896-023-00582-y
27. Khattar, V., Upadhyay, S, & Navarro, R. (2023). Young adults' perception of breadcrumbing victimization in dating relationships. *Societies*, 13(2). https://doi.org/10.3390/soc13020041
28. Durvasula, R. (2015). *Should I stay or should I go: Surviving a relationship with a narcissist*. Post Hill Press.
29. Durvasula, R. (2015). *Should I stay or should I go: Surviving a relationship with a narcissist*. Post Hill Press.
30. Northrup, C. (2018). *Dodging energy vampires: An empath's guide to evading relationships that drain you and restoring your health and power*. Hay House, Inc.
31. Durvasula, R. (2015). *Should I stay or should I go: Surviving a relationship with a narcissist*. Post Hill Press.

CHAPTER 2

1. Oxford University Press. (2023). Hiraeth. In *Oxford Dictionaries Premium English*. Retrieved August 18, 2023, from https://premium.oxforddictionaries.com/definition/english/hiraeth
2. The word "Babyshka" (бабушка) in Russian refers to a grandmother or elderly woman.
3. Perez. G. (Creator). (2001-2002). *O clone* [TV Series]. Rede Globo.
4. Naychuk, O., Kushnerev, S. & Al-Mualla, V. (Program Creators). (1998 to present). *Wait for me* [TV series]. Channel One Russia.
5. Churkin, O. (Director). (1981). *Mama dlya mamontyonka* (translation by author: *Mom for mammoth*) [Animated Short Film]. Soyuzmultfilm.

CHAPTER 3

1. Merriam-Webster. (n.d.). Steadfast. In *Merriam-Webster.com dictionary*. Retrieved August 18, 2023, from https://www.merriam-webster.com/dictionary/steadfast
2. Frank, S. (2020). *The queen's gambit*. Flitcraft Ltd; Wonderful Films.
3. *(Newsletters Translated from Russian to English by the Author.)* "Иногда проигрывать полезно." Газета.Ru. (2013, August 31). https://www.gazeta.ru/sport/2013/08/31/a_5618293.shtml; Дина Аверина: "каждый раз надо завоевывать себе имя заново." ЦСКА. (2019, June 24). https://cska.ru/news/15566.
4. Robbins, M. (2017). *The 5 second rule: Transform your life, work, and confidence with everyday courage*. Savio Republic.

CHAPTER 4

1. Merriam-Webster. (n.d.). Epiphany. In *Merriam-Webster.com dictionary*. Retrieved August 18, 2023, from https://www.merriam-webster.com/dictionary/epiphany
2. Names and all identifying details have been changed to protect the privacy of people involved.
3. Rakovec-Felser Z. (2014). Domestic violence and abuse in intimate relationship from public health perspective. *Health Psychology Research*, 2(3), 62-67. https://doi.org/10.4081/hpr.2014.1821
4. Phelan, M. (2019). The history of "Hurt people hurt people," from pastors to strippers to hustlers. *Slate magazine*. https://slate.com/culture/2019/09/hurt-people-hurt-people-quote-origin-hustlers-phrase.html.
5. Joel, S., Macdonald, G., & Page-Gould, E. (2017). Wanting to stay and wanting to go: Unpacking the content and structure of relationship stay/leave decision processes. *Social Psychological and Personality Science, 9*(6). https://doi.org/10.1177/1948550617722834
6. This dialogue reflects the author's recollection of events, using previous communication and documentation means. All identifying characteristics have been changed to protect the privacy of those depicted. Dialogue has been re-created from memory, electronic communications, digital media, and keeping contemporaneous records.
7. This dialogue reflects the author's recollection of events, using previous communication and documentation means. All identifying characteristics have been changed to protect the privacy of those depicted. Dialogue has been re-created from memory, electronic communications, digital media, and keeping contemporaneous records.
8. This dialogue reflects the author's recollection of events, using previous communication and documentation means. All identifying characteristics have been changed to protect the privacy of those depicted. Dialogue has been re-created from memory, electronic communications, digital media, and keeping contemporaneous records.
9. This dialogue reflects the author's recollection of events, using previous communication and documentation means. All identifying characteristics have been changed to protect the privacy of those depicted. Dialogue has been re-created from memory, electronic communications, digital media, and keeping contemporaneous records.
10. Judith, A. (2004). *Eastern body, western mind: Psychology and the chakra system as a path to the self.* Alchemy.
11. Winters, L. A., & Pierce, J. P. (2018). *The awakened woman's guide to everlasting love.* Sacred Existence.
12. Strong, R. (2022, June 26). *Toxic femininity, explained—plus tips to overcome this mindset.* Healthline. https://www.healthline.com/health/mental-health/toxic-femininity.

CHAPTER 5

1. Merriam-Webster. (n.d.). Lamentation. In *Merriam-Webster.com dictionary*. Retrieved August 18, 2023, from https://www.merriam-webster.com/dictionary/lamentation
2. While this quote is often attributed to Bob Marley, the exact source is unknown.
3. This dialogue reflects the author's recollection of events, using previous communication and documentation means. All identifying characteristics have been changed to protect the privacy of those depicted. Dialogue has been recreated from memory, electronic communications, digital media, and keeping contemporaneous records.
4. This dialogue reflects the author's recollection of events, using previous communication and documentation means. All identifying characteristics have been changed to protect the privacy of those depicted. Dialogue has been re-created from memory, electronic communications, digital media, and keeping contemporaneous records.
5. Kreager D.A., Felson R.B., Warner C., & Wenger, M.R. (2013). Women's education, marital violence, and divorce: A social exchange perspective. *Journal of marriage and the family, 75*(3): 565–581. https://doi.org/10.1111/jomf.12018
6. Names and all identifying details have been changed to protect the privacy of people involved.
7. Merriam-Webster. (n.d.). When it rains, it pours. In Merriam-Webster.com dictionary. Retrieved December 11, 2023, from https://www.merriam-webster.com/dictionary/when%20it%20rains,%20it%20pours.

CHAPTER 6

1. Cambridge University Press & Assessment. (2023). Forelske seg. In *Password Norwegian–English Dictionary*. Retrieved August 18, 2023, from https://dictionary.cambridge.org/dictionary/norwegian-english/forelske-seg
2. Chapman, G. D. (2014). *The 5 love languages: The secret to love that lasts.* Moody Publishing.
3. Chapman, G. D. (2014). *The 5 love languages: The secret to love that lasts.* Moody Publishing.
4. Chapman, G. D. (2014). *The 5 love languages: The secret to love that lasts.* Moody Publishing.
5. Names and all identifying details have been changed to protect the privacy of the people involved.
6. Kozlowski, L. (2020). *Trauma bonding.* Escape the Narcissist.
7. Carnes, P. (1997). *Betrayal bond—Breaking free of exploitative relationships.* Health Communications, Inc.

CHAPTER 7

1. Merriam-Webster. (n.d.). Serendipity. In *Merriam-Webster.com dictionary*. Retrieved August 18, 2023, from https://www.merriam-webster.com/dictionary/serendipity
2. Murphy, R. (Director). (2010). *Eat, pray, love*. Columbia Pictures.
3. Byrne, R. (2006). *The secret*. Atria Books/Beyond Words.
4. Byrne, R. (2006). *The secret*. Atria Books/Beyond Words.
5. Names and all identifying details have been changed to protect the privacy of people involved.
6. Bretherton, I. (1992). The origins of attachment theory: John Bowlby and Mary Ainsworth. *Developmental Psychology*, 28(5): 759–775. https://doi.org/10.1037/0012-1649.28.5.759
7. Abdul Kadir, N.B. (2017). Insecure Attachment. In: Zeigler-Hill, V., Shackelford, T. (eds) *Encyclopedia of Personality and Individual Differences*. Springer, Cham. https://doi.org/10.1007/978-3-319-28099-8_2025-1
8. Simpson, J. A. (1990). Influence of attachment styles on romantic relationships. *Journal of Personality and Social Psychology*, 59(5): 971–980. https://doi.org/10.1037/0022-3514.59.5.971
9. Simpson, J. A., & Rholes, S.W. (2017). Adult attachment, stress, and romantic relationships. *Current Opinion in Psychology*, 13: 19–24. https://doi.org/10.1016/j.copsyc.2016.04.006
10. Dunham, S. M., & Woolley, S. R. (2012). Creating secure attachment: A model for creating healthy relationships. In *Poisonous Parenting* (pp. 81-98). Routledge.
11. Thomas, K. W., & Kilmann, R. H. (1974). *Thomas-Kilmann Conflict Mode Instrument (TKI)* [Database record]. APA PsycTests. https://doi.org/10.1037/t02326-000
12. Thomas, K. W., & Kilmann, R. H. (1974). *Thomas-Kilmann Conflict Mode Instrument (TKI)* [Database record]. APA PsycTests. https://doi.org/10.1037/t02326-000
13. Thomas, K. W., & Kilmann, R. H. (1974). *Thomas-Kilmann Conflict Mode Instrument (TKI)* [Database record]. APA PsycTests. https://doi.org/10.1037/t02326-000
14. Schwartz, R. C. (2021). *No bad parts: Healing trauma & restoring wholeness with the internal family systems model*. Sounds True.

CONCLUSION

1. "Navīna ātman" can be loosely translated as "renewed self." "Navīna" is a Sanskrit term with meanings including "new," "fresh," and "young"; see Sanskrit Dictionary. (n.d.). Navīna. Retrieved August 18, 2023, from https://www.sanskritdictionary.com/?q=nav%C4%ABna. "Ātman" is a Sanskrit term with meanings including "the individual soul," "self," and "essence"; see Sanskrit Dictionary. (n.d.). Ātman. Retrieved August 18, 2023, from https://www.sanskritdictionary.com/?q=%C4%81tman

www.ingramcontent.com/pod-product-compliance
Lightning Source LLC
Chambersburg PA
CBHW072151200426
43209CB00052B/1111